Your Secret to the
FOUNTAIN OF YOUTH

What they don't want you to know about

HGH

Human Growth Hormone

James W. Forsythe, M.D., H.M.D., and
Earlene Forsythe, R.N., M.S.N., A.P.N

MW01492537

FOREWORD

Suzanne Somers

Jim and Earlene Forsythe wallop a resounding grand slam with this pivotal book, destined to serve as an essential anti-aging health guide for many generations to come.

These widely respected medical professionals have won well-deserved praise for their integral work in ensuring that the public can receive injectable human growth hormone.

As chronicled step-by-step in this breezy, informative and easy-to-read guide, injectable bio-identical HGH can delay or even stop impacts of the aging process.

You can start benefiting now thanks to the Forsythes' dogged determination and efficient work. Finally, here, you have found the ultimate users guide for those seeking necessary details in using legally prescribed HGH in a natural and safe anti-aging regimen.

The documented, true-life saga of the Forsythes' battle against bogus criminal charges by the federal government makes this story even more compelling.

A novel by best-selling author John Grisham based on the Forsythes' saga certainly would fly off bookshelves at lightning speed. Yet here, you get all those details first-hand, straight from those who endured our government's horrific prosecution attempt.

Throughout our nation's history, pivotal leaders have fought tough and diligent battles to preserve your rights and freedoms. Everyone from Presidents Washington and Lincoln to Betsy Ross, Clara Barton and Abigail Smith Adams played integral roles in protecting the lifestyles we can enjoy today, many working behind the scenes.

As many of you might know, for a number of years I have been an advocate of bioidentical hormone replacement therapy. Without question, the Forsythes reign among the medical professionals who have played an integral role in this vital process.

With little doubt, you should consider the Forsythes among these pivotal personalities in fighting to meet your needs—even if you have never heard of them until now. Their positive legacy is likely to endure, for reasons you'll soon discover in the pages that follow.

—Suzanne Somers, TV star, author & popular media personality

"Your Secret to the Fountain of Youth ~
What they don't want you to know about HGH"

Century Wellness Publishing
521 Hammill Lane
Reno, NV 89511

Designed by Patty Atcheson-Melton, Wow Design Marketing, Inc.,
&
Margie Enlow, NuDirections Graphic Design Marketing

Forsythe, James W
Forsythe, Earlene

ISBN: 978-0-9848383-0-1

CONTENTS

Avoid high-fat foods

Take recommended minerals

Take anti-aging Vitamin supplements

Add the latest supplements to your anti-aging cocktail

Dedication

To our children, Marc, Michele, Lisa, Pompeo and Sarah,
And their children—our grandchildren—Kiley, Clayton,
Teson & Previn

May their lives be enhanced by our work.

Acknowledgments

This book became possible thanks to the dedicated assistance and encouragement of our entire office medical staff.

Publishing, editing and marketing experts also performed significant roles. Reno Rollé, Lynn Rollé and Bill Gladstone envisioned and eventually developed this publication. Transcriptionist Diane Comstock became crucial thanks to her keen ability at fact checking, while reviewing integral medical terminology.

For their support and dedication, credit also goes to Dr. Burton Goldberg, the "voice of alternative medicine," Joseph E. Brown of Perfect Balance, and Albert Sanchez, Ph.D, of AMARC, Inc.

Patty Atcheson-Melton, along with her partner Margie Enlow, employed their exceptional creativity, patience and persistence in generating this book's cover and layout image. Editors Wayne Rollan Melton and Nancy Padron helped put this entire project together in a cohesive form, in order to ensure that readers learn essential aspects of our personal story and vital medical information integral to "Your Secret to the Fountain of Youth."

Professional guidance and endorsement credit is given to the American Academy of Anti-Aging Medicine. Special thanks also go to "rock stars" in A4M, including Robert Goldman, M.D., Ronald Klatz, M.D., Ronald Rothenberg, M.D., and Mark Gordon, M.D.

About the authors

James W. Forsythe, M.D, H.M.D.

James W. Forsythe, M.D., H.M.D., has long been considered one of the most respected physicians in the United States, particularly for his treatment of cancer and the legal use of human growth hormone. In the early 1960s, Dr. Forsythe earned his M.D. from the University of California, San Francisco, before spending two years residency in Pathology at Tripler Army Hospital in Honolulu. After a tour of Vietnam, he returned to San Francisco and completed an internal medicine residency and an oncology fellowship.

Today in Reno, Nevada, Dr. Forsythe maintains a conventional medical clinic, the Cancer Screening and Treatment Center, and a homeopathic practice, Century Wellness Clinic. A former associate professor of medicine at the University of Nevada School of Medicine, Dr. Forsythe has conducted numerous original clinical outcome-based studies on many natural substances.

For more than 20 years, he has been interested in integrating alternative and conventional medicine.

Earlene Forsythe, R.N., M.S.N., A.P.N.

Ms. Forsythe has worked in the medical profession for 37 years. She received her Master's of Nursing and Nurse Practitionership Degree from the University of California, Davis. She has worked side-by-side with her husband of 32 years managing his integrative medical oncology practice.

In 1998, she became the Health Freedom lobbyist in the state of Nevada. In 1999, Nevada passed the Health Freedom Resolution to promote integrative medical choices in the treatment of chronic and terminal illnesses. Ms. Forsythe represents the voice of health freedom to promote integrative medical choices in the treatment of chronic and terminal illnesses.

Ms. Forsythe represents the voice of health freedom for cancer patients. She promotes integrative therapies in the health health care mangement of these patients'diseased.

In 2000 and 2004, Ms. Forsythe served as chairman of the Republican Party in Washoe County, Nevada, and Chairman for the Nevada Republican Party.

Editor's Note:
Other than in the foreword section, throughout the text of this book, all references to the first person "I," "me" and "my" refer to James Forsythe, M.D., H.M.D., and a vast majority of references to "us" "our," or "we" refer to the co-authors, both Doctor Forsythe and his wife, Earlene Forsythe, R.N., M.S.N. & A.P.N.

INTRODUCTION

Clinical studies indicate that the legal use of injectable bio-identical human growth hormone has the power to halt or even slow the aging process. Also known as HGH, this natural substance causes no harm to people when prescribed in proper doses by a medical professional.

Yet the U.S. Food and Drug Administration, huge pharmaceutical companies and the mainstream medical industry tried to shut down my efforts to tell the world about these conclusions, and to prescribe HGH to patients. Justice prevailed in 2007 when a 12-person jury found me innocent of bogus, trumped-up federal charges alleging that I illegally prescribed HGH.

Imagine my sense of relief when soon afterward, under the sponsorship and auspices of the Food and Drug Administration, the verdict opened the door for me and other physicians to expand the use of HGH for age-related deficiencies. In fact, authorities eventually appointed me to develop the official Food & Drug Administration (FDA) national protocol for how physicians administer HGH.

Through publication of this book, today we're beginning a worldwide crusade to tell you the truth about the many benefits of this amazing natural substance, heralded as a "miracle drug." We feel motivated by an urgent sense of responsibility to tell everyone that HGH—when used under proper medical supervision—can treat numerous medical conditions, and increase the quality of life during mature years, while making you look and feel younger.

Despite government attempts to prevent you from discovering the many benefits of HGH, we're taking a strong stand by encouraging the prescribed, medically supervised use of this essential hormone. Many standard-medicine physicians undoubtedly will become upset that we're divulging the truth here, because in some instances when using

HGH consumers might find themselves needing these physicians' services less.

Through the years, we've discovered that a vast majority of physicians who dislike integrative medicine fail to tell you these vital details. And what you can find in other books on these controversial HGH-related issues is almost non-existent.

Many people admit surprise when we tell them of numerous other uses for HGH, ranging from the treatment of morbid obesity, preoperative and postoperative wound care, severe sports injuries, traumatic brain and spinal cord injuries, and specific types of heart problems, including cardiomyopathies, chronic fatigue, obstructive sleep apnea, and more.

During the year immediately following the trial, I gave numerous speeches to prestigious gatherings of medical professionals, always receiving standing ovations. For the first time many respected physicians nationwide began taking a serious look at HGH as a treatment option. But why is this turnaround finally happening?

Remember that age-old saying, "Information is power." Now that we're spreading the details, people from all walks of life including medical professionals are starting to reach their own conclusions about HGH or in some instances to consider its application for the first time.

Encouraged by these responses, and bowing to steadily increasing public demand since the trial, we decided to write this book to correct the many misconceptions and to get the truth out once and for all. You'll learn why huge pharmaceutical companies and the conventional medical industry tried—with the backing of our federal government— to close our office, put me in prison, and ruin our reputations.

The pharmaceutical industry, often dubbed as "Big Pharma," would love to suppress the information you're about to review. How much money will the mainstream medical industry lose as the use of legally prescribed HGH increases in popularity? If you're no longer suffering from memory loss while enjoying greater vitality, improved organ functions, and increased libido, would you have less need to visit a standard-medicine physician and for drugs such professionals prescribe?

Many people admit they're stunned when learning blow-by-blow details of my arrest and the failed attempts to prosecute me. Like those jurors, you'll discover that our government wrongly used its full power and might in a horrendous attempt to shut down my medical practice.

Just like the jury did, you'll learn the basics of HGH in easy-to-understand terms. Where is the vital substance found in nature, how is it produced, and why do we need it to grow as children and later as adults to maintain our youthful vigor?

Going a step further, you'll learn how to determine if you might be a potential candidate to use HGH. Once you suspect that's the case, it's important to know how to find a qualified physician who can give you a proper and reliable diagnosis, determining whether your treatment or therapy could include injectable bio-identical growth hormone (HGH).

Of course, you'll also need many specifics including: potential costs; whether insurance companies help patients pay such fees; how-to basics on the usual course of therapy; and info on potential minor side effects.

Most important from the view of patients, what specific results should you expect or hope for when receiving prescribed injectable HGH? How much younger will you look and feel, if at all? What about your energy levels, memory, overall organ functions and life expectancy?

All along, you'll probably want to know the pros and cons of using HGH. We'll warn you of what fear-mongers or a traditional-medicine doctor is likely to tell you about this issue. In a no-holds-barred manner, you'll learn how our research and conclusions can shoot down many or all of these bogus arguments in a flash.

First off, as you begin this journey of discovery, we would like to congratulate you for deciding to read this book. Perhaps you have a friend, associate or relative who has benefited from prescribed HGH. Or, maybe you've been lured by the controversy that began soon after this book's release.

We often see a shocked expression flash across people's eyes when first telling them flat-out this undeniable truth: "HGH is not a steroid, but rather a natural substance that reaches its highest concentration in our bodies in our young-adult years." All along, we're seeing widespread public confusion between HGH and anabolic steroids. Simply put, anabolic steroids can cause serious side effects, symptoms never suffered by people who receive legal, permissible doses of HGH.

The mainstream news media clutter about sports heroes using steroids contributed to a widespread misconception that HGH is always considered an illegal substance. Once we get past such misunderstandings, it's time to concentrate on vital basics.

Is there a point in life when it's too late to start receiving injectable bio-identical HGH? Why do humans produce less of this substance as we grow older, resulting in the signs of aging—everything from increased body fat to wrinkles, brittle bones, memory loss, chronic fatigue and graying hair?

In order to understand the answers, you'll first need to know how and why our bodies produce HGH, plus a biological triggering mechanism that gradually slows the natural production of this substance beginning from our mid-20s to early 30s.

From the start, you'll need to keep in mind the basic benefits that HGH provides almost all of us during our childhoods and young adult years. This hormone gives young adults all the physical attributes that many people consider as "youthful."

We all know this means strong muscular bodies, smooth, tight faces, lightening-fast memories, quick reflexes, the capability of running or moving at a rapid pace—plus the ability to heal fast.

But why does the body's natural production of HGH taper following our young adult period, decreasing at an increasingly rapid rate as we edge into our mature years? And from the standpoint of overall health, why do some people seem to age more rapidly than others?

As you find out more about HGH, you'll discover the intricacies of how such biological mechanisms work in the miracle of life. At this point in the learning process, many older people reach what they describe as a joyous discovery when they get legal prescriptions for this amazing hormone.

Imagine the exhilarating feeling of having your quick memory return as your body regains its youthful strength. Think of the reactions you'll receive when people tell you, "Wow, you look so young. How do you do that?"

Indeed, many of our patients happily report such reactions on a regular basis. Vowing their eternal gratitude, they thank us for giving them a new zest for life as their bodies respond to this natural substance that I prescribed.

Part of us wants to respond by saying, "Don't thank us. Thank Mother Nature." Most of the time, we simply allow each patient's physical response to HGH to do all the talking for us. And, of course, as with almost any type of treatment, specific results vary among patients.
On occasion, people ask us if we inject HGH into our own bodies. We

always give the honest answer, "Yes," to the amazement of people who view us as 10 to 15 years younger than our actual ages. Under the care of another physician, we each began receiving HGH several years ago. Our clinic has issued similar prescriptions to numerous celebrities who report similar positive results. You'll soon review the testimonials of everyone from everyday citizens.

Our zest for life, productivity and overall activity levels rival those that I enjoyed during the 1960s and early 1970s. That's when we worked non-stop as students, and as budding medical industry professionals. Every day, we're grateful for the many benefits HGH provides to us and our mature patients who receive the substance as part of their prescribed treatments. Many of these people urge their acquaintances, friends and relatives to get similar prescriptions.

Yet due to a sharp increase in demand, some potential patients must wait a substantial period of time in order to book an initial visit to our alternative medical office, the Century Wellness Clinic in Reno, Nevada. Even many of our regular office visitors are surprised to see the parking lot crammed with vehicles, many with license plates from as far away as New England, Alaska and the Deep South.

Lots of patients make the long trek to our West Coast conventional medicine facility, Cancer Screening and Treatment Center, for treatment that does not entail the use of HGH. A steadily increasing number of visitors are people hoping for prescriptions of this substance. Some patients are East Coast residents who pop into Reno amid business trips to the West Coast.

As you'll soon discover in detail, laws vary widely nationwide on who can prescribe HGH. For instance, a physical fitness trainer in a certain state might be committing a felony if he or she gives or administers injectable HGH to a client. Yet in the same state a doctor of homeopathic medicine can prescribe the substance without raising an eyebrow.

By now you probably sense—and rightly so—that we feel a responsibility to give strong opinions on issues such as this and other controversies involving HGH. What uniform criteria, if any, should be enacted nationwide? How can a person naturally increase his or her HGH levels without having the substance administered? At what point is it appropriate to issue prescriptions?

Delving further, we're eager to give our assessment of why so-called mainstream physicians and non-medical practitioners have locked horns on the HGH issue. Some doctors are likely to balk at our assessment of why the FDA waited until my criminal case to establish protocol for the diagnosis and distribution process.

As the Baby Boom Generation pushes through its middle-age years and into senior status, it's essential for the public to gain a far greater understanding of these issues. Our effort to educate people will take on increasing importance in the coming months and years, as physicians make more discoveries about the many benefits of HGH.

To her credit, my wife, Earlene, stood tall throughout this horrible ordeal, serving as a solid foundation that made our quick bounce-back possible. As the future generations pass, much of the credit for spreading the positive word about HGH must go to this vibrant woman blessed with the most infectious laugh that many people say they've ever heard.

Some of the other positives that emerged from the trial include the solid friendship that I have instinctively developed with our attorney, Kevin Mirch. Within a short span, Kevin became like a brother, a sibling that I never had until he began representing me. We speak at least once daily, his advice and encouragement always golden.

Collectively and individually, Earlene and Kevin stand by me—and beside you as well—in ongoing efforts to enable the public to learn what "they" don't want you to know about human growth hormone.

When word of this book first began to spread and arrangements started for me to appear on the talk-show circuit, I felt struck by a great, satisfying feeling that I had beaten our federal government at its own game. Kevin argued vehemently on my behalf while calling the government's efforts wrongful prosecution. The jury issued an innocent verdict after less than a few hours of deliberation.

We feel humbled and honored when people call us "heroes" for getting the word out, for pushing past the media clutter. Some folks even started labeling us as courageous, dogged fighters, and people willing to step forward with strong opinions—something no one else from our profession seemed willing to do amid the heat of controversy.

Yet we scoff at such labels, for the true "hero" here is not any person, but actually the natural human growth hormone.

Yes, herein rests details likely to change your life for the better, as you proceed down a lifestyle path lined with HGH-filled fountains, the way Mother Nature intended.

--James W. Forsythe, M.D., H.M.D.

Editor's Message

Just about everywhere I go, people inquire about some of my most famous clients. People often ask, "Who are the celebrities you've written or edited for?" and "What is that person really like?" As a ghostwriter and editor for popular media personalities, everyday consumers, corporations and institutions, I have worked with many diverse people in creating or editing manuscripts for several dozen books.

Here's where I'll let you in on a so-called big scoop, one that compelled me to write this foreword for "Your Secret to the Fountain of Youth." Of the widely known clients I've worked with, Doctor James W. Foresythe and his wife, Earlene, are by far the most down-to-earth, everyday folks. They happen to reign as superstars in the medical industry.

For several years, the couple has consistently drawn huge crowds and standing ovations when attending and speaking to homeopathic and standard medical conventions nationwide. Many of the industry's most seasoned health industry professionals appreciate the couples' ground-breaking innovations, plus the fact they beat the federal government and won when fighting for your right to legally use a natural youth-giving substance.

Despite the Forsythes' numerous successes in recent years, perhaps you haven't heard of them until now. Largely as a result of this book, I'm confident they're on the verge of becoming household names nationwide, if they have not done so already by the time you received this ground-breaking publication.

During an eight-month period when we worked on a regular basis in the development of this project, I saw first-hand that the doctor and his wife, a widely respected nurse practitioner and medical administrator, each live with gusto and charisma. While the doctor

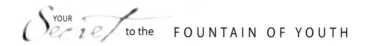

energizes people with his soft-spoken magnetism and gently intense eyes, Earlene mesmerizes everyone with her bubbly voice and bright, positive aura.

My wife, Patty—a widely acclaimed graphics designer—and I have known the Forsythes for many years. Before I met Patty, she already had been friends with Earlene for quite a while.

Individually and together, the Forsythes are like "people you've always known," tantamount to old college buddies, or long-lost relatives, or a favorite uncle and aunt—or just plain good friends. Anyone who has ever become close to people with this kind of spark and gentle intensity realizes how comfortably such magnetizing and nurturing personalities fit into your life, almost as if you've known them since early childhood.

From the days we first became friends as couples, I had always assumed that Doctor Forsythe was my age, with Earlene a bit younger than us guys. Well, imagine my surprise and literal shock when I finally asked the doctor his age, while launching the initial editing work on his book.

"You're what!" I proclaimed—stunned—when he told me. Sure enough, at age 70 the doctor is 18 years older than I, quite a shock to my senses since I thought we were close enough in years to be brothers—rather than a father-and-son separation in age. The secret, he confessed, hinged on the "Secret to the Fountain of Youth." This naturally occurring substance is more commonly known as human growth hormone or HGH, the primary subject of this book.

I became stunned to learn that Earlene is a bit older than me as well. The Forsythes have been using legally prescribed injectable HGH almost daily for several years. Once these details sprang forth, questions began to flow from me almost as fast as I could think of them: How is the substance legally acquired? Where can I get some right away? And what are the side affects?

Fascinated by compelling details from the doctor's initial manuscript of this book, I told him that I had been upset and confused when the government arrested him on bogus charges a few years earlier. At the time prosecutors falsely claimed that he had illegally distributed or prescribed human growth hormone.

"I knew from the moment I first saw those headlines that you were innocent," I told him. "I told Patty that morning that this must be 'some sort of frame-up job,' for we knew that you—Doctor Forsythe—never would have committed the type of horrific crimes that the government charged you with."

Well, about six months following the innocent verdict, after reviewing the doctor's compelling initial draft of this book, I began to learn much more about the Forsythes' vibrant pasts. Both blessed with stick-to-itiveness and gumption since childhood, each overcame separate challenges from early life before eventually emerging together as perhaps the country's leading advocates and champions for the legal use of prescribed HGH.

The basic details of their lives—individually and together as a couple—struck me as so compelling that I joined the ranks of those who insisted that that this book start with the history of their lives, rather than merely chronicling the many benefits and uses of HGH. Once these details are presented, the so-called magic of the hormone and the significance of the Forsythes' huge accomplishments come into clear focus.

More fascinating than a fictional character

From the start, you should know—at least from my view—that in a sense Doctor Forsythe is sort of a modern-day Forrest Gump, except in a much different sense. You might recall Gump, portrayed by Academy Award®-winning actor Tom Hanks in a blockbuster 1994 movie named after the title character.

Blessed with extremely good luck despite his low IQ, Gump stumbles through much of the last half of the 20th Century—becoming a Vietnam War hero, before interacting with that era's revolutionary hippies and meeting some of the world's leading personalities.

Paradoxically, while en route to becoming perhaps the world's leading champion of Your Secret to the Fountain of Youth, in many ways Jim Forsythe engaged in lots of the same activities and accomplishments as the fictional Forrest Gump. The primary difference between Forsythe and Gump becomes evident when you discover that the future doctor employed his keen intellect as opposed to the movie character's relatively low intelligence.

Besides becoming what I consider a Vietnam War hero just as Gump had done, Doctor Forsythe took a fairly similar route in lifestyle—treating a world-renowned celebrity while a medical intern, in this case Gen. Douglas MacArthur. As a young man, Jim also helped several other new doctors in launching a famed medical clinic in San Francisco's Haight-Ashbury District near the peak of the free-love hippie generation of the late 1960s.

"Throughout Doctor Forsythe's career, he has always been right on the edge of where he needs to be—for his patients, and for advancements necessary in the medical industry," said Valerie Marioni, B.S.N., manager and administrator of the Forsythes' patient facilities. "He has never been afraid of facing fear, and there isn't anything positive that he has been unwilling or unable to learn—especially in matters that help his patients."

From Marioni's perspective, Dr. Forsythe's keen mind and vast intelligence—coupled with an accommodating personal style—have enabled him to make significant advancements in medicine, while earning the well-deserved respect and admiration of patients.

"His mind conceives something positive or a specific medical development, and then his heart makes him believe that he can make those advances happen," Marioni said. "Most of the time his ideas invariably become reality for that very reason."

As a child, the future Doctor Forsythe attended a full-time, live-in boys' school—tantamount to an orphanage—because his divorced mother could not afford to care for him. During the years after his release from the school at age 7, through his teenage years, in a sense he became a father to his own mother—at least so it seemed, managing everything from the payments of household bills to grocery shopping.

For her part, Earlene persevered as well, literally the offspring of mobsters and bordello operators. As a young woman, Earlene strived to better herself in joining a respectable profession. While a young adult, she made a four-hour commute several times a week from Nevada to her native Golden State of California—in order to become the first certified nurse practitioner in the northern part of the Silver State.

The birth of a man who changed the medical industry

Born in Detroit, Mich., on Aug. 11, 1938, James W. Forsythe entered the world as the son of an alcoholic father and a hard-working mother, Ruth, a high school graduate who had a stable upbringing. Torn by apparent conflict sparked by the father's penchant for liquor, the couple separated before their only child reached age three.

Through childhood, the future physician heard rumblings that his father had been the black sheep of his family, a rebel and a maverick. The elder Forsythe had earned a reputation as "someone who likes to party and date with dancing girls who performed at their theater in the hotel," owned by little Jim's grandparents.

"All of this temptation apparently was too much for my father," Doctor Forsythe says today, adding that his dad at least had attended the University of Michigan at Ann Arbor although never graduating.

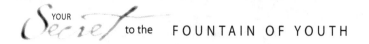

After dropping out of college, the elder Forsythe had worked various finance industry jobs involving banks, trust deeds, stocks and bonds. But the Great Depression ruined Jim's father financially.

The elder Forsythe developed a drinking problem following bankruptcy, the start of a lifelong battle against alcoholism. Well into his adult life, the younger Forsythe—the future doctor—never spent more than part of a single day with his dad.

"I never really got to know the man," says Doctor Forsythe, a senior in medical school in 1964 when his dad died from heart failure at age 69.

Adult mentors inspired the future doctor

Who had inspired the younger Forsythe as a child and later as a young man to excel and achieve, eventually into a position of prominence in the medical industry—where he could reveal "Your Secret to the Fountain of Youth?"

The answer might rest largely in the example set by his mother, Ruth. Her perseverance through dogged hardship served as a model for his character. As a youngster, Jim's inspiration also came from several adult mentors, primarily school teachers and coaches during elementary school and as a teenager.

When Ruth was a young adult, her father—Jim's maternal grandfather—railroad engineer William Brownlee, died of an apparent heart attack. William had gone to sleep on a living room couch after dinner one evening but never awakened. The death shattered Ruth's dreams of attending nursing school.

In subsequent years Ruth's mother, Wilamina, suffered a series of disabling and incapacitating strokes, forcing the young woman to care for the family matriarch along with the services of nursing aides. Lacking alimony, child support or welfare, Ruth worked two late Depression-era jobs to support her son and mother.

Persistent financial hardship and work obligations forced little Jim's mother to place him at age three into a residential group home for boys run by "Nursey," another single parent. More than six decades later, the doctor remembers Nursey as a caring, extremely health-conscious woman who embraced an ardent belief in health foods, from juicing to daily cod liver oil.

"These traits may have had an influence on my own medical career, as they definitely left an impression on me at the time," the doctor says today.

As a child, he stayed at Nursey's on weekdays. The boy spent weekends with his mother, who used this as quality time for excursions to the park or theater with him.

Ruth's mother died at age 77 in 1943 when Jim was five years old. Soon afterward, severe financial hardship forced his mom to place him in a full-time German-Lutheran boys' home in Detroit. The doctor remembers this as a "very strict place to live" for 80-100 youngsters, ages 5-15.

"I remember the male attendants carrying sticks to swat kids who were misbehaving," he said. "We all lived in fear of being swatted, and so we tried to be on our best behavior at all times. I do remember many fights occurring on the playground amongst the older boys. I tried to stay clear of these, and being only five, I was seldom involved in altercations."

Conflict at the boys' home intensified even more when children and adults from the Detroit area were angered by the facility's name as a

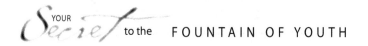

German-Lutheran boys' home amid World War II. These protestors yelled expletives outside the complex, and threw stones at the building or into the playground.

Undoubtedly, these early life experiences helped instill within the future doctor a keen survival technique, the same personal characteristics that enabled him to persevere through trying times and eventually to become a champion of HGH as an adult.

When the war finally ended in 1945, Ruth placed her son in a summer camp where the doctor remembers having "the time of my life" as he learned to swim. An even greater milestone occurred during that period when Ruth married "Proctor," a middle-aged tool and dye maker whose first wife died of cancer.

Ruth and Jim moved to East Detroit into the home where Proctor and his 16-year-old son, Carlton, already lived, an all-white middle class neighborhood. For the first time, Jim lived in a neighborhood with children his own age who never had to endure the types of hardships he had to endure. Many of these neighbors became friends for years to come.

At school Jim excelled in most classes, especially history and social studies. Although occasionally a bit of a prankster who endured his fair share of visits to the principal's office, he found solace in school activities and loved his teachers.

Difficult times resumed

Ruth and Proctor separated and finally divorced following a stormy relationship. The husband had become occasionally mean, grouchy and difficult to live with due to carryover depression caused by memories of his late wife's terminal illness.

Once again Ruth and Jim were on their own, without child support, alimony or welfare, amid moves to Northern Michigan and Chicago. While working several jobs to make ends meet, Ruth rented a home before subletting rooms to older men to augment her income. Forced to mature fast, young Jim took charge of cleaning and meal preparation.

He helped boost their income more by working several afternoon and evening paper routes, also working in supermarkets and delicatessens as a box and delivery boy. Increasingly industrious, Jim plunged himself into studies at middle school, where teachers became his surrogate parents and tennis became a lifelong passion.

Earlene entered the scene

The future love of Jim's life, Earlene Marie Marion, was born when he was 10 years old approaching his 11th birthday. Shortly after an earthquake registering 4.5 on the Richter Scale rocked San Francisco, Earlene was born in that city on March 9, 1949.

Earlene's parents named her in honor of her father, Earl, the grandson of a former mafia-connected family member who ran illicit ventures in the Monterey and Carmel areas of the Central California coast. Well before Earlene's birth, her paternal grandfather changed his surname to Marion from Marioni to escape the mob stigma.

The other side of Earlene's family had an equally unsavory past. During her formative years, relatives confided in the child that her maternal great-grandmother had been a madam in a San Francisco "sporting house" or bordello. Since childhood, relatives attributed Earlene's colorful, buoyant personality and aggressiveness to these genes.

Along with an older sister, Earlene's maternal grandmother, Sadie, had run away from her family's home at age 12 in the early 1900s to escape an abusive father. The siblings traveled to Hollywood in

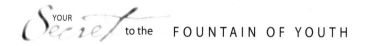

Southern California to seek their fortunes in the silent picture industry. Sadie landed a few bit roles in silent films,

Sadie's life took a dramatic change at age 16 when a 30-year-old man from Norway saw her on Hollywood Boulevard, considering her "cute" in stiletto high heels and bright curly red hair. They married after a short courtship in Venice, Calif., but their first child—a boy—died in childbirth. Their second child, Earlene's mother Beverly, was born in 1930.

Blessed with a deep, sensual voice, Sadie landed work as a cabaret singer. But the young crooner's husband ran off with her best friend, leaving the entertainer without financial support and the responsibility of raising Beverly.

So, little Beverly's aunt—Sadie's sister—often cared for the youngster for weeks at a time amid the singer's busy performance schedule. These included stints as a Depression-era USO entertainer and singer in a Hollywood nightclub, right off the famous intersection of Hollywood and Vine.

At age three, Beverly became attached to a black fox terrier, "Wimpy." The pet never left her side, making life seem at least somewhat bearable when Beverly would need to walk from home to visit stores or attend nearby schools. Beverly would bring home and care for animals that became her only buddies.

Beverly's father neglected to contact the teen during her adolescence in the 1940s, as he failed to financially support his ex-wife and child.

Earlene enjoyed a vibrant heritage

A sawdust and icehouse industry worker for many years, Earlene's paternal grandfather, Earl Marion Sr., retained a real love for music and entertainment. A short, robust man blessed with many raw talents, during the Roaring '20s, he headed a small band that played Bay Area parties, weddings and nightclub gigs. Earl and his wife, Blanche, lived in San Francisco's 21st Street Sunset District in a house that had belonged to her parents.

Impressed by his diverse abilities, neighborhood residents proclaimed him the "Mayor of Irving Street" between 19th Street and 21st Street. Earl Sr. visited shop owners on Saturday mornings to whistle their favorite tunes, tell jokes he learned the previous evening in nightclubs, and to help proprietors greet their customers.

At a little miniature horse merry-go-round in front of Bocoks Mercantile Store on 19th Avenue as a young man Earlene's grandfather greeted parents and urged mothers to put their children on the ride. Then, he gained their admiration by paying the nickel for the rides. Needless to say, Earl Sr. became the person to watch at family dinners and holiday celebrations.

Drawing persistent, endless rounds of laughter from relatives and party-goers immediately before and during the Great Depression, he would put socks over his own ears before making sounds identical to the dog next door—barking feverishly till all the neighborhood's dogs started howling. He possessed an uncanny ability to mimic many diverse sounds, from the whinnies of race horses to the precise tones of musical instruments. Many people liked his trombone the best.

Earlene's father suffered chronic illnesses

Blanche suffered chronic illness from tuberculosis, which she passed on to Earl Jr. during his birth in the late 1920s as the Marion's only child. They lived most of their lives in San Francisco's Sunset District, a short walk from Golden Gate Park.

Despite his illness, Earl Jr. developed into an athlete during his teens in the 1930s and early 1940s, earning a high school letter in swimming.

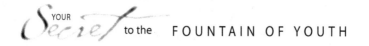

The young man enjoyed constructing model airplanes and cars, plus sailing San Francisco Bay.

After purchasing a small sail boat, he also became interested in messenger pigeons—enough to build a two-story pigeon coupe in his parents' backyard. Every weekend as a teenager, Earlene's father entered the birds in San Francisco coastline pigeon races. Along with fellow high school chess enthusiasts, Earl Jr. formed a club that held tournaments in front of his family's house on 21ˢᵗ Street.

Although an average student, Earl Jr. excelled in math and physics, telling relatives much later that he decided to avoid higher education because his father—Earl Sr.—insisted that he stay in the family sawdust business.

Nonetheless, at 18, he enlisted in the U.S. Marines near the end of World War II, but contracted pneumonia shortly after basic training. He got a medical discharge without compensatory disability payments following hospitalization and a slow recovery. The illness emerged as an apparent blessing in disguise while his unit went on to fight some of the war's most infamous battles including Iwo Jima and Guadalcanal.

Earlene's parents married after a brief courtship

While still in his teens, before establishing himself in a profession and as his lung-related illnesses persisted, the younger Earl met Beverly on a blind date, and they married soon afterward.

A San Francisco physician handled Earl Jr.'s follow-up care, diagnosing the young man with scrofula, a form of tuberculosis that affects the lymph nodes—causing massive enlargement of these organs in the neck and lung. The physician admitted Earl Jr. to a tuberculosis sanitarium ward at San Francisco General Hospital, isolated from other TB patients.

Hospital regulations prevented Earlene and her older sister, Karen, two years her senior and born in 1947, from in-person contact with their father, who remained under quarantine for three years. Relatives and nurses only permitted the children to wave at him through a window, and the sisters usually had to wait outside in the family car.

Beverly's mother Sadie, the former silent film actress and cabaret singer, helped rear the girls during this period. Meantime, during Earl Jr.'s hospitalization, physicians filled his lungs with oxygen in an archaic attempt to keep tuberculosis organisms from growing; at the time, there were few effective antibiotics for treating pulmonary tuberculosis.

Earlene's life transition kicked into gear

When physicians finally discharged Earl Jr. after several years, he took his small family to Tacoma, Wash., where he attempted to attend college to become a minister. But soon afterward, Tacoma doctors admitted him to a tuberculosis sanitarium in Washington state after he suffered a setback. Once again, medical regulations prevented the girls from seeing their father for several years.

The children lived in near-poverty conditions as their mother and grandmother each worked part-time jobs, as supplemental welfare covered living expenses. When doctors finally discharged Earl Jr. a second time, he got a draftsman job with the San Francisco power company—earning a decent salary. The family's lifestyle finally stabilized, and they bought a home and a car for the first time.

Earlene attended Jefferson Elementary in San Francisco, the same

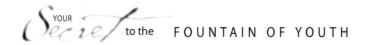

school her father had attended. But fire destroyed the building after a sixth grade student committed arson; the destruction forced officials to send its students by bus to various local schools.

This setback failed to prevent Karen and Earlene from enjoying numerous outdoor activities with their family, like kite-flying at San Francisco Marina, biking in Golden Gate Park, and watching their father play football with his buddies near the city's famed Cliff House on the Pacific Ocean shore.

Beverly became a Blue Bird counselor for her daughters within the Camp Fire Girls of America organization, also serving as its head San Francisco Area counselor. Earlene and Karen learned to sew in Camp Fire Girls programs—skills the mother and her adult daughters would later use in making family wedding dresses and bridesmaids outfits.

A continual succession of moves began

More than two decades before meeting Earlene, life took a different track for Jim at age 15 in 1953 when he and Ruth packed their black 1949 Mercury for a cross-country trek and moved permanently to Los Angeles.

Ruth landed a legal secretary job and they found an apartment between Hollywood and Glendale, close to Marshall High School—which Jim attended three years until graduation, his longest stay at any institution during his upbringing.

They lived in a beautiful, affluent neighborhood near Griffith Park where he often visited the nearby Riverside tennis courts. During this period he started to write a book, "Raising Ruth," but never got beyond the first chapter.

"It was all about my experiences raising my mother and being more of a father to my mother than she was a mother to a son," he recalls.

"I handled the finances and the housework, and oftentimes the meals while she worked."

During that first summer Jim's many jobs included landscaping, as well as an industrious, mega-energetic carpenter's helper. The teenager managed to play all three years for his school's varsity tennis team— which won a league championship thanks largely to his athleticism.

While earning straight A's in high school, Jim grew to love his teachers and tennis coach as they became his surrogate parents. He became much happier than during his early difficult years.

Just as important, during Jim's junior year in high school he met a schoolmate's father, Doctor Emery, a cancer surgeon. That physician became what Jim remembers today as "the best role model I had ever seen. He was an impressive, stately man with an erect posture and a professional bearing. I idealized being just like him someday. I had no other male role model in my family. So, much of my appreciation for him was at a distance."

Inspired, Jim worked as a part-time orderly at nearby hospitals, gaining a rewarding sense of fulfillment, the position a perfect fit with his personality while helping helping sick and disadvantaged patients.

Meantime, his congregational minister, Alan Hunter, an intelligent, knowledgeable and kind man, became a close friend and mentor. Jim kept busy during summers, mowing lawns while also working as a stock boy in various department stores. By now the industrious, ambitious teenager had honed the hard-working ethics that would enable him to becoming a champion for using HGH in later life.

Scholastic achievements launched success

On the strength of excellent grades in high school, Jim won a scholarship to the University of California at Berkeley in the San Francisco Bay Area right after high school graduation at age 18 in 1956. At the time, the university was an Ivy League-style school, where men wore khaki pants and loafers, while women donned knee-length plaid skirts with cotton, collared shirts and camel-hair coats.

With the aid of several scholarships, Jim maintained a 3.6 grade point average while working several jobs for the necessary extra tuition—a lengthy list of jobs that would have made even the industrious President Teddy Roosevelt pale by comparison. Jim's many positions included sorority house manager, sorority hasher, pharmacy assistant, postal worker, short order cook, department store stock boy, furniture sales person, kitchen manager and many other positions.

As if all this weren't already enough, during summers he worked as a firefighter, children's camp counselor, dance instructor, tennis teacher and even as a gold mine worker in Alaska. But perhaps the most memorable job was serving as a personal aide and chauffeur to Henry J. Kaiser Jr., heir to the Kaiser Health System fortune.

Today, the doctor remembers the position as a well-paid job that "gave me a taste of being the first au pair physician to an industrialist of great wealth." The medical industry magnate even promised Jim a position upon graduation as an administrator or medical professional at one of Kaiser Health System's hospitals.

Kaiser suffered from multiple sclerosis. Part of Jim's work involved giving this employer personal care in his Oakland Hills area home. Jim often guided Kaiser through personal therapy sessions, before chauffeuring this man to the Kaiser Health System Building on Lake Merritt in Oakland.

At the time, the young Forsythe owned only two suits. Reflecting back, he admits that, "I did my best with different shirts and ties to make it look like I had a lot more clothes—when, in fact, I was extremely poor. I did my best with my limited wardrobe to look the part of an assistant to the wealthiest man in Oakland."

Continually curious and energetic, Jim's favorite classes included American poetry, sculpturing, comparative embryology, organic chemistry and physiology. Perhaps most of all, he loved intellectual debates—commonly called "bull sessions"—in the residential men's homes.

Jim's medical school studies soon followed

Upon graduation from undergraduate studies in Berkley in 1960, Jim married Joan Fisher, a former high school classmate in Southern California; they had attended the senior prom together.

Understandably proud of his achievements, Jim earned his undergraduate degree in physiology from what later became known as "the last normal class from the University of California at Berkeley." It wasn't until several years later that he returned to campus amid the anti-war, radical and revolutionary hippy era; by then the formal Ivy League attire and atmosphere had disappeared.

On the strength of Jim's continued good grades, his admittance applications were accepted at both the University of California at San Francisco Medical School and McGill University in Canada.

During the fall of 1960, Jim and his new bride moved into a walk-up, one-bedroom apartment in the Haight-Ashbury District of San Francisco as his medical schooling and career began. Unaware that within a few years their neighborhood would evolve into a haven for hippies and drugs, each day he made the one-mile walk to and from the medical school campus on Parnassus Hill.

Today, the doctor remembers gross anatomy as a mandatory, unpleasant initiation into the world of medicine. During medical school studies Jim used knowledge learned as an undergraduate to his advantage,

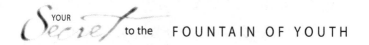

earning an appointment to teach physiology to his new classmates—generating much-needed extra income.

In January 1961, one year after Jim entered medical school, he and Joan had their first child, Marc. The birth became the first live delivery witnessed by many of Jim's classmates. Determined to support his budding young family while completing medical school, he worked from 6 o'clock each evening to 6 every morning as an on-call, seven-day-a-week registered laboratory technician.

During this four-year period through medical school, Jim worked a wide variety of diverse jobs, such as doing heart surgery on dogs for research labs, serving as an orderly in local hospitals, and as an extern in various hospitals to complete medical histories and physicals on newly admitted patients.

Always bright and curious, despite his seemingly non-stop, 24-hour work and study schedule, Jim's medical school courses seemed to get easier to him as the years progressed. For elective studies, he managed to team up with doctors in various specialties and sub-specialties, working with them in local and rural hospitals for one- and three-month periods.

Earlene moved to Reno from San Francisco long before Jim

The year after Jim entered medical school, in 1961, Earlene was 12 years old as she moved with her family to Reno, Nevada—where her grandparents Sadie and Jerry found a home. The new Nevadans convinced Beverly and Earl Jr. that Reno would be a perfect place to rear the children, largely due to the region's snow skiing and diverse outdoor sporting activities.

Soon after moving to Reno, Beverly found jobs as a keno runner at the Harold's Club and Harrah's casinos, and also worked as a car hop without roller skates at a drive-in restaurant.

While handling these many jobs, Earlene's mother also returned to school to earn a Licensed Practical Nurse or LPN certificate. Saint Mary's Hospital in Reno admitted Beverly to its a nursing program; Beverly worked there after graduating, the beginning of a 30-year career.

While Earl's tuberculosis remained in remission, he held a regular job as a draftsman for Reno-based Sierra Pacific Power Company and took correspondence classes to earn an engineering degree.

Throughout the early 1960s, Earlene excelled in her middle school studies while developing talents in gymnastics and swimming. After high school graduation in the late 1960s with a 3.5 grade point average, Earlene entered the University of Nevada, Reno, where she majored in nursing sciences. She earned a scholarship from a "doctors' wives" organization, the Auxiliary to the Washoe County Medical Society.

Volunteering as a candy striper at Saint Mary's Hospital, Earlene worked her way through school doing part-time jobs such as a nursing assistant and ward clerk at the facility—plus babysitting. While a sophomore and senior working for Richard H. Licata, PhD, an anatomy professor, she was in charge of cadavers donated to the university.

Earlene assisted the professor in preparing his practical exams for students. She helped them conduct the professor's research on mammalian heart cells, specifically the coronary arteries and the heart muscle's rhythmicity and conductivity.

At age 20 in 1969, Earlene enlisted in the Army with three other nursing students, including Karen Mingus and Patricia Fagan. Shortly after the women visited a recruiting station, Earl Jr. received an unexpected

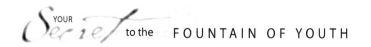

call from an Army recruiter asking: "Mr. Marion, did you know that your daughter just joined the Army Nursing Corps as a private first class?"

Earlene's father became horrified that his daughter might be going to Vietnam, a prospect which never materialized. During Earlene's junior year at the university she met William DeRay Lombardi, a legendary football player, rodeo bull roper, lumberjack, cab driver, pest exterminator and crop duster.

The administration lowered the boom

The future doctor's usual non-stop work and study activities took a different course, when administrators unexpectedly summoned him to the dean's office during his junior year. Making it clear this wasn't a disciplinary matter, school officials asked Jim how he would be able to complete his final two years without substantial financial resources.

Challenged, Jim explained that he was working every moment possible, nights and weekends, and that he definitely would meet his goal of working his way through the final two years of medical school. His explanation satisfied school officials, who allowed his studies to continue.

Despite Jim's bravado, he began to worry about how he would be able to finance his expensive education. So, as a solution, he turned to the U.S. Army's new medical school program, which promptly commissioned him as a second lieutenant and put him on a pay grade during his senior year.

In exchange, Jim owed the military three years of service, beginning when his internship ended. Perceiving this as a "light at the end of the tunnel," Jim cut back on his night and weekend work and moved with his family into a second-story flat adjacent to a park in San Francisco's fashionable Richmond District.

The couple's second child, Michele, was born in March 1964 during Jim's senior year. Fortunately, right after he graduated a few months later, the military placed him at Letterman Army Hospital at the Presidio less than two miles from the family's apartment.

Despite having a dependant wife, two children and countless part-time jobs off and on, Jim graduated in the top 19th percentile of his class. He might have been the only student who needed to take advantage of the Army's program.

Rotating medical internships were the vogue after Jim graduated; he took every type of medical study available other than pediatrics, which he felt never suited his temperament.

While enjoying all his various internships—as noted earlier—at one point he was able to see the legendary Douglas MacArthur, General of the Army, as a patient in a private room. Age 84 at the time and within one year of his death, the general was very ill. Jim noticed the general wore a copper bracelet and inquired about it. The general answered, "I've worn this many years for my arthritis."

Mid-way through the internship, the commander of Letterman Army Hospital summoned Jim to tell him that the institution's administrators had learned he was moonlighting in local hospitals during his off hours.

"This is illegal under Army regulations," the commander told Jim—ordering him to cease and desist immediately. Taking this seriously, Jim quit his externship at a local private hospital in San Francisco.

War emerged as a factor

The Vietnam War had heated into a full-fledged major military conflict by the time Jim's internship ended in 1965. Still unsure what specialty to spend his life practicing, for the time being he decided to enter a pathology residency—considered an excellent background for almost any internal medicine or surgical sub-specialty.

As Jim leaned toward a possible career in internal medicine, various surgical practices remained options including obstetrics-gynecology, urology, or ear-nose-throat surgeries. He ruled out psychiatry, avoiding the possibility of having to listen to neurotics, depressives and psychotics up to eight hours daily.

When Jim finished his internship at the Presidio, the Army sent him along with the rest of his internship class to San Antonio, Texas, for a four-week basic medical training course, a combination of military school and field work.

Right when training ended, President Lyndon B. Johnson spoke via closed-circuit TV to the men, who gathered in an auditorium. Johnson told these physicians that as newly trained doctors they would be welcomed in South Vietnam immediately as U.S. military forces escalated there.

"Needless to say, I was happy to be going into a pathology residency in Hawaii, rather than into this more sobering alternative," the doctor says today.

By this point, he had been promoted to captain at a higher pay grade, enabling him to move his young family into off-base housing—which the young couple considered a "dream come true in paradise."

Jim's increased earnings enabled him to buy a home on the windward side of the island, near beautiful Kailua Beach. Little Michele and Marc went barefoot, bodysurfed and sailed in a small Sun Fish™ craft which Jim purchased for his family.

Despite their lives in this tropical paradise, Jim decided that giving the military three years of service for every one year of training would force him to commit as a 20-year regular Army Medical Corps officer—not what he wanted for a lifetime career.

Jim decided that a lifetime in pathology was out of the question. He preferred to deal with people rather than laboratories and autopsies. For the short term, he had two options—either tell the Army he wanted a transfer to the mainland to complete his payback period, or volunteer for a one-year tour of duty in Vietnam.

Following a period of tortured soul searching, he finally decided to proceed with his standard six-year payback period. Soon after telling the military his decision, the Army transferred Jim to Fort Bragg, N.C., to join the 82nd Airborne as assistant chief of pathology at the large Womack Army Hospital.

Hippies and the power of love

While en route to North Carolina from Hawaii for his newest assignment, the sights and sounds of San Francisco during 1967's "Summer of Love" emerged as an eye-opening experience. The once-sedate and rather quaint Haight-Ashbury district where he had lived with Joan while attending medical school had become the center of the hippie movement's universe.

Either stunned or perplexed, Jim watched the streets fill with barefoot, tie-dyed hippies amid the persistent aura of marijuana. For him, it was an unbelievable revelation of how much the world had changed in just a few years, amid growing animosity against the military and its involvement in Vietnam.

While in San Francisco for this limited period, Jim seized the opportunity to work for several days at the famed Haight-Ashbury Free Clinic. A former classmate, Dr. David Smith, founded the clinic on

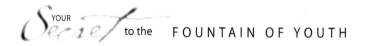

June 7, 1967, to treat drug-related problems and sexually transmitted diseases among free-loving hippies.

Along with several of their classmates, David and Jim started the small storefront medical operation. The facility received national recognition during the counterculture revolution of the 1960s.

Personal and social transitions progressed

Later that summer Jim drove his young family cross-country to Fayetteville, N.C., where he assumed his assignment as assistant chief of pathology at Womack Army Hospital. While at Fort Bragg, he developed respect and admiration for the U.S. Special Forces units comprised of dedicated young soldiers—many who had already served in Vietnam.

Soon afterward, Jim earned his next promotion, this time to major. Along with his family, he spent the next 18 months enjoying the glorious fall and spring seasons of North Carolina. Partly because homes were inexpensive compared to Hawaii, he and Joan purchased a comfortable three-bedroom house on a ¾-acre lot with pine trees. Building a tree house for the couple's two children became his first priority.

In April 1968, the military sent Jim to Washington, D.C., for a postgraduate pathology training course. Within hours after the class ended, Jim and Joan got caught in a huge traffic jam, amid rioting that ignited following news that the legendary civil rights activist, the Rev. Dr. Martin Luther King Jr., had been assassinated in Memphis, Tenn.

Within hours of the killing, Washington became an armed camp, the military sending tanks along Pennsylvania Avenue to protect the White House and the Capitol Building. The skirmishes forced the couple to scrub their plans to dine out in Washington that evening before seeing a play at the famed Ford's Theater.

Seven months later, in November 1968, Jim received orders that he had feared for some time, a directive that he go to Vietnam in January 1969. Prior to this, he had been given the option of going to Germany for three years—an assignment requiring an additional three years of payback. Instead, he decided to take his chances on a one-year Vietnam tour that would complete his payback requirement.

"I had already made up my mind to leave the military and return to civilian residency training in another specialty," Jim recalls. "The temptation of a tour in Germany—while attractive—was not something I wanted to undertake because of my long-term career plans.
"

In preparation for the move in November 1968, Jim moved his wife and two children to Los Angeles, where they could live near his in-laws for a good family support system during his year-long absence.

During a one-month leave from the military in December 1968 immediately prior to Jim's scheduled departure for Southeast Asia, he landed a temporary job as a general practitioner in Los Angeles in order to brush up on his diagnostic and prescription skills.

Following tearful goodbyes with his family in early January 1969, Jim spent a few quality days with his mother, Ruth, and her fifth husband, Harold. On the appointed day, the couple drove Jim to Northern California's Travis Air Force Base, where he climbed aboard a 707 aircraft packed with sweaty, smelly soldiers from across the U.S.A. for the 17-hour flight to Saigon, then the capitol of South Vietnam.

From the view of Valerie Marioni, the manager of Forsythe's offices today, in many ways his decision to go to Vietnam showed the same type of courage that he still maintains in his allopathic and homeopathic medical practices.

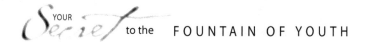

Jim witnessed horrific death and destruction

Ground fire from enemy forces greeted the aircraft as it approached Tan Son Nhat Air Base near Saigon, resulting in a 30-minute delay as friendly forces fought off Viet Cong rebels who hoped to bring down a plane filled with new GIs.

"After deplaning I felt like kissing the ground, because I had arrived safely," Jim said.

Crews unceremoniously piled the passengers' duffel bags behind the aircraft after the plane taxied to a barricaded area off to one side of the runway. Commanders sent the men to get personal supplies at a relocation center. There, officers told the men that each soldier would be deployed to various areas within South Vietnam within three to seven days.

During this boring and tedious delay, the soldiers spent 24 hours a day playing cards, drinking beer and smoking—while teling bad jokes and complaining about the Army.

On the third day, Jim received orders to report to the 93rd Evacuation Hospital in Long Binh, 30 miles north of Saigon, exactly one year after that facility had been opened. Military personnel placed him in a new two-story barracks within hours after he arrived—just in advance of the annual Tet celebration of the Vietnamese New Year—that nation's most important holiday.

One year earlier, the Viet Cong had launched an eight-month military surge, called the Tet Offensive because it began in the early morning hours of the holiday, Jan. 31. During the well-coordinated 1968 campaign, 80,000 Viet Cong troops hit more than 100 towns across the country.

A second Tet Offensive began the day after Jim arrived, when incoming rocket and mortar fire lasted one week. Sirens blared around the clock, and U.S. commanders told all personnel at the 93rd Evacuation Hospital to find the nearest bunker and stay put. Jim and other replacements who accompanied him to the hospital had not yet been issued weapons.

"Had the base been overrun with Viet Cong, we would have pretty much been on our own," Jim said. "My first exposure to death in war came as I witnessed a second lieutenant laying dead on the ground just outside a bunker, having been hit by mortar fire before he could get to the bunker for safety."

Along with several other unarmed officers, Jim crawled into a 5-foot-wide aluminum drainage tube that went under a highway. Holding a blanket and a few rations, he spent several nights there—awakening each time an explosion came close. After this military surge faded within days, officers sent him to his assigned hospital, where he promptly became the stand-in chief of pathology.

Due to increased casualties caused by the second Tet Offensive, Jim became the area's only forensic pathologist. As a result he got the inglorious job of performing autopsies on American soldiers.

"Aluminum caskets were piled as high as the ceiling in the autopsy room," Jim said. "As soon as a body was brought in, it was my job to make proper identification and, through a limited autopsy, describe the cause of death by entry and exit wounds—or the blast injuries, or the fire injuries, or by any other cause of death."

Although sometimes the cause of death became obvious right away, on other occasions the reason was initially unknown. Surviving soldiers had pulled many of the young bodies from warm swamp water where the corpses had been rotting for days. Many of these remains were ballooned up, green and foul-smelling.

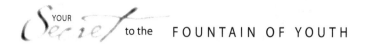

"This 10-hour-a-day, unpleasant ordeal was mine alone," Jim said. "No other pathologist was assigned to the hospital."

Standard procedure required Jim to perform dental checks and look for scars or other identifying tattoos, because some bodies had become unidentifiable.

"It's difficult to comprehend the horrors that Doctor Forsythe and others on his military team must have endured," Marioni said. "A lot of people—a vast majority of us—probably would never have been able to accomplish what he did in Vietnam, and every since then as well.

"In all aspects of life, he has shown fortitude and bravery. His many accomplishments have gone well beyond the scope of what would have been expected of him, in both his career and in his personal life. He's always so concerned for his patients that he often forgets about any concerns for himself."

Fortunately, thanks partly to Jim's higher rank of major, in February 1969 a replacement came for the position. Commanders promptly sent Jim further north to the 312th Evacuation Hospital at Chu Lai, in the southern portion of the I-Corps. He served as chief of pathology there while simultaneously holding a similar position for a surgical hospital 10 miles away in the jungle.

Tranquility intermixed with bombardment

This latest Evacuation Hospital sat on the shores of the South China Sea, away from front-line battles and much quieter as a result. Using his rank of major, he took a second-floor walk-up room, 20 yards from a steep, 100-foot cliff with a view of the azure blue waters and a coral reef 100 yards offshore.

During their brief breaks from duties, doctors and nurses navigated a steep trail to a sandy beach, where they enjoyed warm water—plus an abundant display of tropical fish at the reef. Via mail, most ordered or received fins, masks and snorkels. Determined to enjoy the setting as much as possible, Jim also ordered a spear gun that he used to harpoon sea bass and other small fish. A mess hall cook prepared these catches for Jim and his friends.

Besides overseeing tropical medicine, blood banking, and malaria-related duties, Jim gave frequent lectures to the staff on various medical subjects. He and other personnel reserved nights for drinking and dancing.

Jim diagnosed various types of malarial infections five to 15 times daily. In the process he discovered that many soldiers purposely failed to take their twice-weekly malaria pills. These men strived to catch the disease so they could get shipped out of the country or have their tour of duty cut short.

Twelve enlisted men of varying ranks comprised his laboratory staff at the two hospitals. Conducting a wide variety of standard laboratory work from urinalyses to routine chemistries, they used universal donor blood in almost all cases—but the blood still needed to be crossed-matched with recipients.

The staff's brazen behavior surprised Jim, especially when most of them openly smoked marijuana during breaks from hospital and lab work. This behavior intensified to the point where the hospital commander lost his ability to discipline them at this time during the war. So, the commander chose to ignore the situation. Vietnamese housemaids often brought marijuana sticks in exchange for Salem® cigarettes because these women preferred menthol from such tobacco.

Overlooking the sea, the officers' club featured a small bar, a dance floor, kitchen and several restrooms. As the social activities center for all officers on the base, the facility proudly displayed a typical '60s slogan above the entry: "If it feels good—just do it!"

Despite the base's apparent tranquility, with the sea on one side and the Americal division on the other, the base sustained frequent, sporadic, round-the-clock rocket attacks—keeping all personnel on edge. Many officers and soldiers wore flack jackets and helmets for much of the day.

The possibility of being attacked from the sea remained remote. U.S. personnel knew the Viet Cong could emerge from so-called rat holes at any time, causing immediate widespread death and destruction in the hospital area before crawling back into their tunnels.

Jim considered the direction and targeting of sporadic attacks as haphazard. From his perspective, an individual U.S. soldier's ability to survive on the base depended on the fate of targeting coupled with varying weather conditions.

"Whenever someone was killed or injured from the rocket attacks, we all knew that it was a strictly random or unpredictable event," he said. "The random attacks caused the greatest fear of all my entire time there."

Those determined to return home alive or uninjured took their own individual precautions. To lessen the probability he would get killed in his upstairs room, Jim surrounded his single-frame bed with sandbags up to mattress level. And he placed a 6-foot piece of corrugated sheet metal—the width of his bed—under the mattress, also placing a similar sheet on the floor beneath the bed.

A distinctive whirring sound warned personnel before an impact or explosion, giving soldiers at least some time to react. Luckily, at least for Jim, no such explosion occurred near the barracks while he was within the compound.

Enemy artillery killed a U.S. nurse

The hospital complex's luck ended a few months later on June 8, 1969, when 1st Lt. Sharon Lane, at age 24, became the first U.S. nurse to die in combat in Vietnam. A thin, shy, dark-haired woman, she had been working a swing shift in a children's ward, sitting on a bed, when a rocket hit the back of the ward.

Hot shrapnel blazed into the lieutenant's right neck, severing the main artery to the brain. Massive hemorrhaging forced the entire blood supply from the woman's body by the time medical personnel could rush her to the operating room.

"I had the sad task of performing a forensic autopsy on Sharon to describe the nature of her fatal wound," Jim said. "The entire camp was in a state of mourning for the next month, and we all realized that the next rocket 'might have our name on it.'"

In mid-July 1969, a single rocket hit a crated-up Cal 30 sailboat that a California yachting company wanted to offer as recreation and rehabilitation services to soldiers. After initially being delivered before this attack, the U.S. naval harbor master had ordered that the vessel remain crated and stored adjacent to the base dental clinic. This officer had been concerned that Viet Cong could mine the yacht at anchor if it were in the harbor.

Weaponry experts estimated the rocket that hit the yacht during the late morning hours had been fired from 10-12 miles away, a direct hit on the uncrated yacht. This attack hit while Jim rode in a Jeep® off base en route to his surgical hospital laboratory. Enlisted personnel with him phoned in to inquire if the hospital had been hit. About 20-30 people in the dental clinic could have been killed if it were bombarded rather than the crate.

Upon returning to base, Jim saw that the yacht had been pulverized to

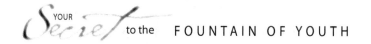

golf ball-size pieces near a hole in the wall of the clinic. All personnel inside escaped serious injury.

Needless to say, Jim began counting his remaining days at the base, as everyone on the complex came to realize that American forces could never muster a clear-cut victory like the USA and its allies achieved in World War II. Americans began to understand that the war might end with some type of stalemate, perhaps similar to the conclusion of the Korean War.

Helicopter crash-lands into the sea with Forsythe on board

Late that year, several weeks prior to Jim's scheduled return to the American mainland, a U.S. Army helicopter crash-landed into the South China Sea with him and about a dozen other American military personnel on board. During the days prior to this crash, he went with several nurses and doctors from the Evacuation Hospital to an island about 35-40 miles east, about the size of Catalina Island off Long Beach, Calif.

Vietnamese refugees, primarily women and children, had gone to this Southeast Asia island to escape day-to-day gun battles and bombings in their homeland. Jim and the other Americans had flown to the island to aid refugees who suffered from malaria, dermatological diseases, infected wounds, dysentery, and other ailments. The Americans spent one day seeing several hundred women and children, dispensing medicines, malaria pills and other stop-gap treatments.

Then, following a late luncheon with male leaders on the island who described themselves as the island's chieftains, the Americans boarded the double-rotor blade helicopter for a return flight back to their base. Red lights flashed on the pilot's instrument panel less than 10 minutes after takeoff, indicating a rotor blade malfunction.

"Take off your shoes and be prepared for an ocean landing," the pilot told everyone after turning around to face the passengers. Jim heard the props slow down noticeably. After turning around, the pilot made it to within 50 yards of the island shore—crash-landing in a shallow area 2-3 feet deep.

His boots and khaki pants off, Jim waded to shore in his underwear along with other medical personnel. Everyone had escaped serious injury. Lacking weapons, the survivors scurried to find any place on the beach they considered safe.

"I was able to bury myself in the sand and some beach reeds, up to my neck and chest, in order to partially camouflage myself," Jim said. "It was unknown to us whether or not there might be Viet Cong on the island who would take advantage of our disabling situation."

The next morning Jim felt lucky to awaken unharmed and free after sleeping through the night. Soon afterward, at 7 a.m., a second U.S. helicopter arrived to retrieve them. This experience made Jim glad his tour of duty would soon end. Since then, he has remained impressed by the simple, uneducated, industrious, hard-working, self-sufficient people of South Vietnam—a society that never benefited from everyday luxuries that Americans take for granted.

Forsythe returned to face new challenges

Rebellious black Americans shouting "black power" delayed Jim's scheduled return flight from the Saigon air base in January 1970. The boisterous soldiers shouted angrily, making hostile remarks to flight attendants and pilots.

"This plane will not be leaving the airport until all rowdy behavior has ceased and until troops begin behaving properly," the pilot told passengers, after entering the cabin to speak to them in a forceful manner. The aircraft suddenly became quiet because everyone wanted to return home. The plane soon landed in Guam, and then Hawaii.

Following a brief stay in the Aloha State to visit longtime friends from his former residency at Tripler Army Hospital, tears filled Jim's eyes when he reached the mainland—landing at Travis Air Force Base in Fairfield, Calif. During debriefing there, officers told the soldiers to wear civilian clothes as soon as possible because anti-military and anti-war sentiments had intensified, particularly in the San Francisco Bay Area.

Although Jim had some personal negative feeling about the nation's involvement in Vietnam and the war's apparent futility, he believed people who showed animosity toward military personnel behaved with supreme disrespect. Jim's heart commanded that he honor those who put their lives on the line or died for our country, rather than burn draft cards or escape to other nations.

After Jim hurriedly changed clothes, his mother and her husband picked him up at Travis. His mom was a nervous wreck after reading that a U.S. military plane had recently crashed after leaving Saigon, prompting her to fear that Jim had died in the accident.

"Her depression lifted immediately when she caught sight of me," Jim recalls. "And her mental attitude became one of equanimity."

Jim spent that night in San Francisco before taking an early morning flight to the Burbank airport, where Joan, Marc, Michele and his in-laws met him in the only celebration he was to have as a returning soldier. The military then assigned him to Letterman Army Hospital on the Presidio in San Francisco, where he was to fulfill his final six months of required duty.

However, at this juncture in their lives, Jim and Joan experienced marital difficulties. Joan stayed with Marc and Michele in Southern California. Jim flew there from San Francisco every other weekend to spend time with their children. His final six months in the Army went by fast as he busied himself, teaching Army residents about tropical medicine and doing daily surgical pathology chores.

During this period, Jim purchased a 24-foot sailboat with his bachelor friend Jack Malmgren, a psychiatry resident. They rented an apartment together to share expenses. On weekends, they sailed to various Bay Area communities including Sausalito and Angel Island.

Following an honorable discharge from the military in June 1970, Jim signed up for ongoing duty in the Army Reserves. Still a major at the time, Jim became convinced that following his seven-year military stint the U.S. would avoid engaging in war anytime soon in the wake of the public outcry against Vietnam.

"I believed the money during my planned upcoming residency would come in handy, especially maintaining two households," he said.

Stanford University soon accepted him for a residency program, and he gained a similar position at Children's Hospital in San Francisco amid a love affair he had with the city at the time. Today, he recalls wanting to become part of the excitement created by the building anti-war movement.

One year later Jim qualified to begin sub-specialty training after completing a required 12 months of internal medicine residency. For the next milestone, he chose to enter a hematology and oncology fellowship at the University of California at San Francisco, which immediately accepted him. This transition created little stress, since

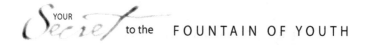

at Jim's alma mater he knew the basic facets of the hospital and its personnel.

In hematology, he specialized in disorders, diseases and organs of the blood, while oncology involved cancers—at the time considered a relatively new specialty, the first year that such boards were offered for certification. A famous researcher, Dr. David Wood, served as director of the Cancer Research Institute where Jim trained.

Within this group, Jim entered an elite group of oncologists, many who went on to become chairmen of various university programs after this post training. As the years passed many of these physicians became what Jim describes as "rock stars" in the field of oncology—Sidney Salmon, M.D., David Golde, M.D., Mike Haskell, M.D., and David Alberts, M.D. Eventually, many of these physicians wrote standard textbooks for the new medical specialty of oncology, literature still used by physicians nationwide for training purposes.

Earlene entered adult life with excitement

Following a short courtship, Earlene and her high-energy, entrepreneurial lover, William DeRay Lombardi, married at the famed Bucket of Blood Saloon in Virginia City, a 30-minute drive from Reno. Her folks became horrified at the notion that she had married a leader of the university's notorious Sundowners' drinking club. An atrophic leg caused by a childhood bout of polio never slowed down DeRay, who held his own in many barroom fights.

Shortly after Earlene and DeRay married, they brought a small casino and bar in the Old West-style town of Austin in north central Nevada. Soon afterward, Earlene became pregnant, and she continued in the Army Reserves as a Second Lieutenant.

Pushing past heartache during this marriage and still striving to better herself, Earlene began her five-hour commute to attend a nursing school in Davis, Calif., to obtain a Master's in Nursing Certificate and to become one of a handful of people in Northern Nevada certified as an Advanced Practitioner of Nursing. Throughout this period, she worked full-time as a cardiac nurse and as a public health nurse.

For her public health duties, Earlene worked in the Sun Valley community north of Reno, following up on child abuse cases to check on youngsters for the Washoe County District Health Department. One memorable case involved an underweight infant living in a run-down trailer with his mother and grandparents. During a baby clinic exam, medical personnel had determined the child was malnourished.

Nine months pregnant, Earlene held a baby scale in one arm and stood on the front porch of the infant's home when an older man came to the front door before she had a chance to knock.

"What are you doing here?" he asked sternly, mistakenly believing Earlene was a social worker there to take the child to foster care. "Nobody is going to take my grandson."
"I'm not a social service worker; I'm a health nurse," she said. "My job is to weigh the child."

Without letting her inside, the man rushed to the back of the trailer, before promptly returning with a shotgun—telling her, "If you don't get the hell out of here I will let you have it."

Earlene ran back to her Volkswagen; momentarily, a shotgun blast ripped into the back of the vehicle, destroying the fender and trunk.

Earlene's family transitions evolved

Earlene and DeRay's first child, Lisa Marie, was born in December 1970 when Earlene was 21 years old and still attending college; their son Pompeo "P.J." arrived in March 1974.

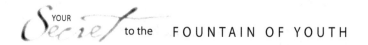

Meantime, DeRay did well financially as owner of the Reno-based Donner Corporation, investing in real estate, but his alcoholism started destroying the marriage. Rather than face the possibility of Vietnam, Earlene worked as a blackjack dealer in their Austin casino. Her parents and grandparents took care of Lisa Marie and P.J. during subsequent years, amid numerous separations and reconciliations between the couple.

Shortly after P.J.'s second birthday, DeRay went to the store to buy bread for that night's dinner. That's when this entrepreneurial father met up with old drinking cronies, and the men ended up traveling to Rio de Janeiro on a whim. DeRay disappeared there for 13 days without a word, not even a phone call to Earlene.

Refusing to submit to DeRay's disrespectful treatment of her, Earlene hired an attorney and filed for divorce. DeRay found his belongings thrown out upon his return, and processors served him with divorce papers soon afterward. Eventually, the couple used the same attorney to dissolve their marriage. They remained good friends until several years later when DeRay died in a car accident.

Jim's interesting life transitions emerged

Still embracing workaholic habits established since grade school, Jim worked at second and third jobs during his training period. Amid his hectic schedule, he worked as Medical Chief of Welfare in Oakland, Calif., and Medical Director in the Women's Hospital in San Francisco. Here in the early 1970s, he saw his first cases of AIDS, well before physicians realized the cause and specifics of the disease.

Within one year after their separation began, Jim and Joan tried to salvage their marriage. She moved with Marc and Michele to Marin County north of San Francisco, where the couple bought a three-bedroom home on a hillside overlooking Mount Tamalpias. Jim took a 30-minute commute to San Francisco, where he found a downtown practice position with two oncologists.

The couple drifted apart during the next two years, before finally deciding to divorce in 1974—one of the most difficult decisions of Jim's life.

"I did know that Joan and I both would eventually be happier with other spouses as our personalities—after 14 years of marriage—did not coincide," Jim said. "In retrospect, this was a wise decision because both of us are happily married at this time, and we both have been for more than 30 years."

Upon divorcing, Jim left the San Francisco oncology practice at Saint Francis Hospital, tired of big city commuting and having to serve on a half dozen hospital staffs. Sensing the need to live and practice in a smaller town, he began considering possibilities throughout the West including northern and southern California, Oregon, Utah, New Mexico and Nevada.

Before long he bought a condominium at Lake Tahoe, lured by his love of snow skiing while also enticed by the middle-town size of nearby Reno, nicknamed "The Biggest Little City in the World." In the fall of 1974, he quit his oncology practice in San Francisco and relocated his practice to Reno, eager to regularly take the four-hour drive to the Bay Area to be with his children.

In Reno, he began practicing with an older physician who—although not a trained oncologist—handled such procedures by default. The community lacked such specialists at the time. This interest by the physician stemmed from the death of his own son, who died of leukemia before his fifth birthday. The longtime Reno doctor happily welcomed Jim as a partner because the field of oncology was just beginning to blossom.

Jim's beginning salary of only $25,000 failed to approach his requirements for alimony and child support, so he took a second job as an emergency room physician, a position he held for two years. This

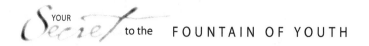

extra stint ended in 1976 when Jim's medical practice became too large for him to handle the additional work while sufficiently boosting his income.

About this time Jim rented an old historic mansion on the Truckee River in downtown Reno, listed on the historic home tour and once the residence of a prestigious state senator. Jim brought few items when moving into the unfurnished residence, partly because he owned few tangible assets then.

Still relatively unknown in the overall region, he took a historic organization's community tour through his own home. As people walked through the house, he heard a woman comment, "Oh, my, they certainly haven't done much with the interior decorating, have they?" The comment embarrassed Jim, although he also considered the observation humorous.

Working as the only oncologist in northern Nevada, Jim drew patients from hundreds of miles away. He found himself rapidly overwhelmed with patients that other doctor's preferred to avoid dealing with, mainly those with advanced stages of cancer.

During the next few years, he fought for and developed cancer wards at the city's only two major medical facilities at the time, Saint Mary's Hospital and Washoe Medical Center. Jim often tended to 30-40 hospitalized patients at any given time, making rounds to visit each of them twice daily.

Largely because the oncology field still was considered relatively new in such small communities, Jim worked as his own chemotherapy nurse without the benefit of a professional assistant to handle such chores. He ordered the pharmaceuticals, mixed them, started intravenous lines and administered these substances himself, all duties normally performed by nurses.

Jim remembers this as a very time-consuming and taxing part of his work, although he enjoyed the chores as the practice thrived thanks to his diligence. Even so, the onslaught of patients needing extensive care played a big role in prompting Jim and the mature physician who recruited him to bring on a third partner.

The medical industry boomed

By this point in the early 1980s, Jim became medical director of the region's first HMO or health maintenance organization. This position angered his senior partner, philosophically opposed to such programs and PPOs or preferred provider organizations. The conflict motivated Jim to go out on his own, in part to a newly built local facility, Sparks Family Hospital—which had constructed an oncology ward for him to operate.

This transition alienated some local physicians who believed the new facility initially failed to meet the community's standards. Some doctors started referring to Jim's referral base as "fall off." Even so, he began enjoying autonomy by having his own oncology ward and serving as its director, operating that division as he deemed fit, in a high-quality manner.

During the following 20 years, Jim entered and left numerous partnerships with professional associates for a variety of reasons, a common practice in the medical industry.

Jim entered a new romance

When moving to Reno, Jim brought along his new girlfriend, Mary. But the relationship fizzled within two years. As he recalls, "because of my busy, time-consuming schedule and frankly my not being able to spend time with Mary, she became disenchanted with our relationship and left Nevada, moving back with her family to Mojave, California."

After the separation, Jim remained active in the Army Reserves, on

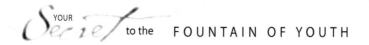

duty one weekend monthly. Upon Jim's arrival in Reno, the military appointed him medical officer in charge of the community's United States Army Reserve Hospital. He became impressed with his nursing staff, particularly Earlene Marion Lombardi, a stunningly beautiful 26-year-old redhead, blessed with smarts and a bubbly personality.

Somewhat later, Jim learned that Earlene had separated from her husband, and she reared their two small children with help from her parents. Right away, Jim became impressed by the fact that Earlene kept working to become an advanced nurse practitioner.

She regularly took a five-hour commute to the University of California at Davis in an effort to earn an advanced practitioner of nursing degree. At the time such courses were not offered in Nevada.

Despite Jim's attraction, he avoided any attempt to date Earlene, preferring to avoid getting involved with someone who regularly underwent separation and reconciliation with her spouse.

"Especially with two children involved, I felt that it was best to let things resolve and then, if she permanently divorced, I would try to establish a lasting relationship," Jim said. "There was no doubt that I was definitely attracted to her and wanted this outcome to materialize without my interference in her current relationship."

Finally, Earlene and her husband divorced in 1976, and she and Jim became engaged later that year. They married a little over one year later in February 1978. Jim became a stand-in father for Earlene's two children, Lisa Marie and "P.J.," ages eight and five at the time.

Jim and Earlene's romance blossomed soon after her divorce from DeRay. The doctor and nurse arrived at a church for their scheduled nuptials on Valentine's Day in 1978, only to discover the building locked without a way to get inside. Rick Kilgore, Earlene's brother-in-law, crawled through an unlocked window on that chilly night, triggering an alarm—but the minister soon arrived to open the doors.

Earlier, Jim's son, Marc, at age 14 had moved to Reno with him on his own volition, while the doctor's daughter, Michele, remained with his first wife, Joan. So, when Jim and Earlene were married, they initially had three children in their home, Marc, Lisa Marie and P.J.

"I am a very lucky man to have found Earlene, who has been the love of my life for the last 30 years," Jim said. "We need each other."

Earlene nearly died

Within months of her wedding with Jim, Earlene suffered numerous miscarriages and nearly died from a tubular pregnancy—losing a quarter of her blood. Physicians gave Earlene more than four units of blood in order to bring her out of shock and stabilize her. Then, doctors performed emergency life-saving surgery at Saint Mary's Hospital while Jim was at a business meeting in San Francisco.

The Forsythes' mutual child, Sarah, was born 16 months after the wedding. The couple hired an au pair from Denmark; this woman moved to Reno, where she cared for Sarah until the child reached two years old. The Forsythes needed the au pair because Earlene spent this period working full-time at the university, plus part-time jobs as an air-flight nurse and as a real estate agent.

Another unforeseen tragedy struck during the early years of their marriage. Earlene's brother-in-law, Rick Kilgore, fell asleep at the wheel and was killed on Interstate 80 near Lovelock about 90 miles northeast of Reno. Kilgore had been driving his wife, Earlene's younger sister, Valerie Marioni—who would become their office manager—and the Kilgore's three small daughters, home to Montana after spending the Christmas holidays in Reno.

Kilgore had awakened as the vehicle spun from the road. He over-corrected the steering wheel, causing the vehicle to spin down the highway and overturn five times. The young father died instantly. His daughters suffered major injuries and Valerie sustained a thrombosis in her leg before a full recovery that left her without major physical problems.

From the accident scene, the girls were sent via air ambulance to Reno's Washoe Regional Medical Center where each underwent surgery. By the time the ambulance arrived at the hospital, Jim had assembled a team of surgeons there to await their arrival.

Beginning two months after the accident, the girls and Valerie lived with the Forsythes and their children for an 18-month period. During that span, Earlene's parents built a home to accommodate them. Then, Valerie and her daughters lived in the new house for five years.

Jim diversified his medical career

Jim became disenchanted with conventional oncology in the late 1980s after starting oncology wards at all three Reno-area hospital

He considered the situation depressing, observing that only a few patients emerged as long-term survivors of more than 3-5 years after suffering advanced stages of cancer. Those lucky enough to survive often had symptoms of toxic chemotherapy, from Chemo Brain Syndrome to peripheral neuropathies.

Chemotherapy also caused cardiac, liver or kidney damage among many survivors. Some suffered chronically low blood counts, requiring periodic transfusions. Still others became endangered by persistent low white blood counts which caused frequent infections. Chronic bleeding episodes occurred when platelet counts dipped to seriously low levels.

"The quality of their lives, even though they had survived cancer, was oftentimes very low, and so I wondered if it was worth the price to pay for survival," Jim said. "There is an old saying in oncology, 'we cured the cancer but the patient died.'

"Since entering the field of oncology, it has often surprised me that there were very few patients of mine—and I can think of only two offhand—who actually committed suicide because of their advanced disease. A cancer patient in general is a real fighter, who will to go to extremes to do everything he or she can to beat the disease."

So, in the early 1990s, while in his early and mid-50s, Jim became interested in finding a niche that would enable him to practice medical oncology in an integrated fashion. Determined to broaden and improve his services, Jim decided to "push the envelope" by becoming a homeopath—enabling him to use both conventional and complementary therapies with cancer patients.

At the time, Century Clinic reigned as the Reno area's largest homeopathic facility, operated by Dr. Katrina Tang and Dr. Yuen Tang, a Harvard-trained standard allopathic physician as well as a world-renowned homeopath. The Tangs eagerly sought to bring another standard allopathic physician into the practice, partly due to problems with Yuen Tang's own health and with federal agencies.

Jim arranged to spend 2-3 hours daily at Century Clinic after completing regular patient duties at his own office. At Century, he saw patients whom the Tangs felt needed some conventional therapy such as standard oncology treatments, or patients outside the Tang's level of expertise.

Jim's prestige and knowledge increased

Jim's part-time work at the clinic continued for about one year, until he arranged to buy Century Clinic from the Tangs. Yuen Tang retired for health reasons, while Dr. Katrina Tang continued practicing there with Jim. Meantime, Jim continued his standard oncology practice operating his longtime business weekdays, 10-12 hours daily.

Jim helped patients whom he felt needed conventional therapies such as chemotherapy, and people deemed suited for complementary homeopathic therapy. This process worked well, the only glitch coming in 1995 when a grandmother of a patient in his 20s complained about the clinic's billing services. She contended that billing for laboratory work was out of line with the area's other clinics.

Yet the grandmother failed to understand that the clinic's bills for laboratory services also bundled fees for the patients' homeopathic medicines. The Medical Board also failed to understand this point; the panel fined Jim $1,000, plus $44,000 for the cost of investigating the woman's complaint, plus expenses necessary for reviewing medical charts and billing practices.

"I would not fight the allegation because I was not yet under the Homeopathic Boards," Jim said. "The ruling by the Board stated very clearly that 'there was no malpractice involved, and there was no inappropriate medical care—but that the billing charges should not be bundled together with the homeopathic medicine charges.'"

Negative media reports about the board's ruling damaged the reputations of Jim and his facility, which he renamed Century Wellness Clinic. Soon afterward, he completed his homeopathic boards, giving him a greater sense of protection. This milestone cleared the way for him to practice as his individual patient's condition dictated

Later, in 2002, Jim and Dr. Katrina Tang decided to split their practices. She talked of retirement or possibly moving back to her native Taiwan. With the help of lawyers and accountants, they separated the practice's assets, while Jim kept the name Century Wellness Clinic and maintained all patient charts.

He then moved the physical part of the clinic into his own building, already the site of his standard allopathic medicine oncology practice, Cancer Screening and Treatment Center of Nevada. Since then, the two clinics have operated under one roof. This is exactly what Jim had hoped for at the beginning of his venture into integrated oncology, engaging in both types of practices at once.

Jim had a variety of medical partners and professional associates over the next three years. Some of these affiliations dissolved due to differences in medical philosophy, or because of the other physicians' desire to practice only conventional oncology. Some transitions with associates took an emotional toll on the Forsythes, ranging from bankruptcies to marital problems or drug abuse among these various professionals.

Even so, together as seasoned business partners and as individuals, the Forsythes persevered and continued to maintain their practice on a high level. This superior degree of professionalism even had continued through the First Gulf War of the early 1990s, when both Jim and Earlene got called to standby for overseas duty.

Finally, in 1993 Jim retired as a full colonel following 26 years of Active Army reserve and National Guard duty, the last 10 years as State Surgeon for these military branches. Earlene resigned as a major after serving as State Nurse for 10 years.

Jim's prestige and philanthropy spread

In 2000, the highly esteemed and nationally respected Dr. Burton Goldberg, often referred to as "the voice of alternative medicine," hailed Doctor Forsythe as the "top integrative oncologist in the country."

Best-selling author Kevin Trudeau, writer of several books on natural treatments, listed the Forsythes' Century Wellness Center of Nevada as "the best cancer clinic for natural cures."

Jim's practice ran clinical outcome-based studies on numerous natural products, including "Paw-Paw" and "Poly-MVA." Jim also developed a unique treatment process called Forsythe Immune Therapy; these treatments included homeopathic supplements and "Glyco-Essentials," in an ongoing study of immune-stimulating therapies.

With far more degrees or certifications than most physicians or medical professionals, by the early 21ˢᵗ Century Jim had become board certified in medical oncology, utilization review and quality assurance—also board eligible in clinical pathology, gerontology and anti-aging medicine. Following successful completion of homeopathy training, he became certified under both the Nevada State Board of Medical Examiners and the Nevada State Board of Homeopathic Examiners.

During the same period, Jim also served on the founding board of Ronald McDonald House in Reno, which allows the families of ailing patients admitted to local hospitals to stay at a nearby home at reasonable rates.

In addition, as if all these duties weren't enough, he served as chairman of numerous medical boards, including the tumor boards, utilization review boards, cancer committees and peer review organizations. Adding to his many responsibilities, he also served as the medical director of five Northwest Nevada nursing homes.

Along with their staff, for a number of years the Forsythes also ran free cancer screening clinics for African Americans and Hispanics. All along, Earlene ran numerous fundraisers for judges and political candidates. She became active in the GOP, becoming chairman of the Washoe County Republican Party and eventually holding a similar position for the Nevada State Republican Party.

In collaboration with Reno Rollé, a widely acclaimed author, business executive, health expert and entrepreneur, Jim co-authored "The Ultimate Guide to Natural Health." Before Rollé became president of Red Rock Pictures, they developed BõKU™ Super Food, a green powder food supplement containing many important vitamins, minerals, herbs and food products. BōKU™ plays a vital role in bringing up the body's pH, when taken regularly for the purpose of helping the body's immune system fight cancers.

The Forsythes solidified their vibrant medical practice

During his 34-year practice, Jim has seen more than 200,000 patients, receiving only one administrative fine from a medical board. His record as a physician remains quite clean. For each cancer patient, he has always offered three standard options:

1. Conventional chemotherapy alone
2. Conventional chemotherapy with complementary therapy
3. Complementary therapy alone

Meantime, Jim developed medical practices or treatment criteria, the latest of which resulted in a 78 percent survival rate among breast cancer patients and a 70-80 percent survival rate among patients who suffered from extremely serious Stage IV cancers. The Forsythe Immune Therapy research involved 300 patients during a 40-month period.

"These results compare very favorably with any statistics in the conventional allopathic literature," Jim said.

In addition, for the Nature's Sunshine Company of Utah, he ran clinical outcome-based studies on Paw-Paw Cell-Reg™, natural twigs from a tree and used as a cancer treatment in people and animals.

Meantime, Jim's second study on Poly-MVA®, hailed as a unique combination of various substances including amino acids, minerals and vitamins, showed a 30-40 percent favorable overall response rate in all Stage IV cancers. This study indicated a five-year overall 32 percent response rate to Poly-MVA®, developed by McKeen-Garnett Laboratories of Long Island, N.Y.

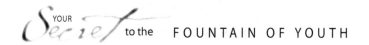

A combination of palladium and alpha lipoic acid, this tightly bound complex product causes cancer cells to get overwhelmed with energy—thereby resulting in the death of these invaders.

A third study that began in June 2005 has involved the homeopathic product salicinum, with a trade name of Salicinium™. When combined with certain immune therapies, this process is called "The Forsythe Immune Therapy." Patients with extremely serious Stage IV cancers were given this as an option, either with or without chemotherapy. This ongoing study has shown some excellent response rates.

Jim plans to eventually present results of this study to the federal Food and Drug Administration as an investigational new drug application or IND, an initial step in getting a new drug approved for prescription use.

"The studies I have done with this supplement show that it has almost no adverse side effects and, therefore, it is a superior product to any chemotherapy on the market," Jim said. "The Salicinium blocks the fermentation of sugar enzymes. When a cancer cell takes up a sugar molecule, the cancer must metabolize that sugar—thereby producing energy molecules through a process called 'anaerobic glycolysis.'"

The inclusion of anerobic glycolysis is the key factor that makes the process safe for all other cells of the body, quite the opposite from the physical ravages inflicted by chemotherapy products prescribed by standard allopathic physicians, a process that extensively kills good cells throughout the body.

Family transitions progressed

Jim's mother, Ruth, passed away quietly in 2002 in a Reno nursing home at age 88 after suffering a fractured hip, following a stroke that left her unable to eat—causing her health to rapidly fade from kidney failure. During the final months before Ruth died, Jim had been able to see her on a daily basis; the facility where she lived is less than 100 yards from his office.

"She did not suffer at the end and died peacefully," Jim said. "However, her death was very hard for me to assimilate, as we had been through very tough times together throughout my tumultuous childhood. Even after her cremation, I still find it hard to spread her ashes in San Francisco Bay, as she had wished. I will do this at a time when all of the children are together for me, on a boat, with appropriate eulogies to her memory."

Ever since Jim and Earlene began courting each other and married, "they've been a dynamite package together," Marioni said. "They compliment each other, enhancing each other's lives in every aspect— from their professional careers to their personal lives. People who get to know them sense this right away."

A driving force in their professional success, Earlene "helps keep the doctor in check, helping him remember to focus on all the important aspects of their hectic lives," Marioni said. "It is often said that 'Behind every great man is a good woman.' Well, as a couple, they prove that's true in every way. She helps motivate him."

During the Forsythes' first several years of marriage, Earlene operated a Lamaze® International business, preparing young parents for childbirth for various Reno-area obstetricians. She also worked at the Veteran's Administration Medical Center, and as an assistant professor in the Health Science Department at the University of Nevada, Reno.

Earlene taught physical assessment skills to pre-med, nursing and physical education students. From 50-75 students signed up for each semester expecting easy-A grades, only to discover her as a stringent taskmaster on their knowledge of the head, neck, heart, respiratory and reproductive systems.

Each semester the sex education block taught by Earlene proved interesting, drawing many non-registered newcomers—as 300 students packed her individual classes. Instruction included playing explicit sexual education tapes.

"During these sessions, not a sound could be heard from any of the attendees," Earlene said. "Many students brought guests who were on the university's various athletic teams."

Doctor Forsythe became a champion of HGH

Besides Jim's groundbreaking work involving HGH, "he's really quite a renaissance man in the area of cancer treatment," said Michael Gerber, M.D. and H.M.D., a homeopath and president of the Nevada Homeopathic and Integrative Medical Association.

"Doctor Forsythe deserves a lot of praise for his courage in renouncing those false allegations against him," said Gerber, of Gerber Medical Clinic and Wellness Center.

The Forsythes' many positive life transitions as a couple and as individuals all lead to the point where the federal government sent a "shill" patient into his office in September 2004—a middle-aged federal agent who stressed the apparent need to use injectable human growth hormone or HGH.

Within the medical industry, Jim emerged as a champion of injectable HGH during the late 1990s and early this century. His intense interest in anti-aging medicine served as motivation to learn everything possible about the hormone. Gradually during this period he began prescribing HGH to patients, but only after medical tests indicated their bodies produced insufficient amounts of the hormone.

Through this process, the Forsythes earned the well-deserved respect of medical professionals and anti-aging experts nationwide, Marioni said.

"Jim's arrest and the government's attempt to prosecute him stunned the medical community," Marioni said. "The news of charges being filed against Jim stunned homeopaths around the country."
On an almost unanimous basis, Jim's patients who use injectable HGH report phenomenal or at least moderate increases in energy—"doing things they've never done before during their mature years," Marioni said. "A lot of physicians might be jealous of this, but they shouldn't be because we're all in this together."

Throughout the ordeal, Doctor Forsythe's professional staff and many of his patients remained committed to him—"always holding faith that he would win, and that justice would prevail," Marioni said. "We knew that what the doctor told us through that period was right on the mark, that all he needed to do was tell the truth in order to get the right verdict.
"The whole time, the entire staff maintained absolute faith in the doctor. We all knew that he had an extraordinary medical practice, and that he had done nothing wrong whatsoever. While remaining supportive, we all conveyed that we truly believed in him. But that doesn't take away from the fact it was a difficult time for all of us."

Marioni recalls that before and during the trial, "When the doctor's patients and people who knew him heard about what was happening, they went into a state of shock saying things like 'I can't believe this happened.' All the people who truly knew Doctor Forsythe and what he does stuck together as a solid, unbendable team."

—Wayne Rollan Melton

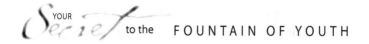

CHAPTER 1

Bang! My attorney and I smashed a government conspiracy

"Is this a joke?" I asked a dozen federal agents as they bolted into my home on a hill overlooking a private lake and downtown Reno, Nevada.

"No," a federal Food and Drug Administration officer barked back at me. "We have a search warrant for money laundering, smuggling, trafficking and introduction of an unapproved drug into interstate commerce and illegal distribution of an unapproved drug."

"Is there anyone else in the house?" yelled one of the agents. They included authorities from the FBI and the U.S. Immigration Customs and Enforcement agency.

"Just my wife," I answered honestly, still stunned by this intrusion, aware she was in the kitchen in another part of our home, cooking fried eggs for our breakfast. Just a few minutes earlier, I had been there with her, when through our large windows she noticed three dark SUVs suddenly appear at the top of our driveway.

"What are those cars doing there?" Earlene had asked me.

"I don't know, but I'll go see," I said, before hurrying down a winding hallway to a back door facing a breezeway that leads to the garage.

I got there just as the intruders prepared to knock the door down with a battering ram. They all wore black flack jackets, and some had stocking caps. After I told them Earlene was there, they demanded to know if I kept guns in the house.

"Yes, I have three pistols in our dressing room," I said, immediately before an officer left to search for and confiscate the weapons.

Treating me as if I were a criminal rather than among America's most respected doctors, one of the agents ordered me to kneel as he pushed a gun to my forehead.

Momentarily, agents intercepted Earlene as she came down the hallway to see what was happening. Horrified, I watched them push a gun against her fleece vest.

Gazing through our front window as the U.S. government invaded our home, I caught a glimpse of my family's 6-foot by 4-foot Old Glory, lightly flapping in a slight breeze from a pole in our front yard.

"Is this really America?" I thought. "What on earth is happening to our country?"

The government treachery emerges

During the difficult few years following that fateful day, February 16, 2005, we discovered that my arrest stemmed from a conspiracy created by numerous federal agencies.

They don't want you to know that prescribed injectable human growth hormone—often called HGH—is perfectly legal. Studies by our clinic and by numerous other medical experts show this natural hormone often hailed as a "miracle drug" can reverse many signs of aging when prescribed and administered in appropriate doses, while causing no adverse side effects.

Through the conspiracy, partly headed by federal prosecutors, I became the first and only physician in United States history to ever be charged with prescribing HGH to a patient for an off-label use as an anti-aging treatment.

Many thousands of physicians and other medical professionals were already giving similar prescriptions. Yet our government chose to single me out for prosecution, perhaps at least in part because many people considered me a fast-rising star in studying HGH and legally prescribing the substance to patients who truly need its many benefits.

On Nov. 1, 2007, a 12-person jury acquitted me of these bogus charges, thereby clearing the way for medical professionals nationwide to continue issuing legal prescriptions for HGH. Yes, beginning as early as this year, you can take steps to legally benefit from this hormone— which many people think of as the equivalent to the Fountain of Youth.

Details the government wants to keep from you

Arrested at age 68 for the first and only time in my life, I sat alone in a county jail cell. Mystified by events that transpired, I took comfort in knowing that I had done nothing illegal. Agents found HGH in the refrigerator of my home, legally prescribed to me by another physician for a legitimate medical condition.

I also felt confident, aware that my clinic's results consistently showed that when administered in mature people, injectable HGH reduces wrinkles, removes unsightly age spots, and re-energizes the libido while reducing body fat and increasing muscle mass and improving cardiac efficiency.

Many patients report a boost in energy, while precise medical tests consistently show decreases in bad cholesterol and a corresponding increase in good cholesterol. Bone density increases, sharply decreasing the probability or risk of severe fractures that a high percentage of mature people suffer.

Little did I know at the time that federal agents and prosecutors were beginning to trash my once-pristine reputation, trying to portray me in the news media as a sleazy doctor who employed questionable techniques. Authorities released me from jail on my own recognizance within one day. But severe damage to my medical practice had clicked into full gear.

During the investigation, some agents told patients never to return to my office. And while searching my clinic amid their probe, investigators actually answered the phones by saying: "Taco Bell"—before telling patients that my practice was under investigation for alleged criminal activity. Agents told callers to "seek medical services elsewhere," and "never return" to my clinic.

As you might imagine, many of our worried or perplexed patients heeded the advice, while others went elsewhere after seeing front-page news stories and TV interviews as various authorities worked diligently to soil my name. During the 14 months immediately before and even after my acquittal, the clinic's patient totals have remained sharply lower than before, particularly due to a sharp decrease in local patients exposed to the publicity.

People died as result of the feds

Worst of all, more than a dozen cancer patients died after being ordered by these agents to stay away from our office. Some of these people were unable to find adequate or comparable care, and in other instances the cessation of treatments put patients off track from returning to good health. Generally, we use standard and alternative medical treatments on my cancer patients, a process that never involves injectable HGH—but rather integrative oncology protocols.

We'll never know for sure whether these former patients would have lived if they continued under our care. But, the overall histories of these patients indicated that many or all of them would have survived.

Complicating matters, before, during and after the trial, I never was told the names of my accusers. And when arresting me, agents failed to read the required Miranda Warning. Prosecutors contended that I had wrongly prescribed HGH to an undercover agent who never needed such treatments.

Yet, at trial, my attorney convinced the jury that I had followed all required medical protocols, except perhaps for failing to order an optional urine test that would have determined if the middle-aged agent's body was producing insufficient amounts of HGH. Even so, before issuing the agent a prescription, I had ordered a required minimum blood test which concluded that the man had inadequate amounts of the vital hormone.

Outwardly, the government prosecuted me in an effort to pursue justice. Yet in reality, at least from our view, the bogus arrest and trumped-up charges stemmed primarily from one overriding goal: to curtail or shut down altogether the legal prescribing of HGH nationwide.

Conspiracy theories abound

We suspect one of our disgruntled former employees may have given authorities false information in an attempt to get revenge because of her dislike for Earlene. My wife's success as Chairman of the Nevada Republican Party had also caused extreme jealousy among political rivals, who may have joined the conspiracy. Earlene had introduced President George W. Bush at political rallies in Nevada during the 2004 presidential campaign, less than six months before my arrest.

Adding a huge log to the proverbial flames, at trial we proved that the lead federal agent who pursued my arrest had previously been reprimanded by his superiors for unprofessional conduct. Was I deemed a "prize," put in the proverbial crosshairs in hopes of reigniting the agent's faltering career?

Cramming high-power weaponry into their cannons, the prosecution called a parade of traditional allopathic physicians who testified that injectable HGH is not a standard part of their acceptable treatment protocol. In a swift and fatal blow to the prosecution, my attorney showed a standard FDA medical book, deemed "a Bible" of sorts, also called the "Orange Book," listing the drug as legal and approved while proving unequivocally that prescribing off-label prescriptions of injectable HGH is accepted and permissible.

At one point, the prosecution even smeared egg onto its own face by delivering to the court boxes filled with injectable HGH, displaying the material as if evidence against me—yet each clearly and fully labeled as having been shipped to the offices of other physicians. So an obvious question emerged: Why was I being singled out while many other physicians continued to obtain and issue off-label prescriptions for this natural and highly effective substance?

Allopathic physicians are taught to avoid issuing prescriptions of natural HGH as an anti-aging measure. Instead, under strict guidelines set by the American Medical Association and the FDA, these doctors issue prescriptions of costly drugs, sometimes for the treatment of aging symptoms, everything from brittle bones to high levels of bad cholesterol. Amazingly, these physicians avoid HGH although it costs much less in treating the same characteristics, while in many instances providing better natural results.

By contrast, many alternative medicine physicians prescribe injectable HGH, and a vast majority of these professionals are not standard allopathic physicians. Well, I'm unique in this regard, practicing as both a standard allopathic oncologist, as well as a licensed practitioner of alternative medicine. Our clinic's results prove that alternative medicines are effective, though allopathic physicians believe much of it is quackery, primarily because we use natural methods such doctors are taught to avoid.

Tied to Big Pharma, mainstream standard physicians have worked diligently to crush or eliminate any public perception that injectable HGH should or will serve as a safe and practical alternative to expensive drugs.

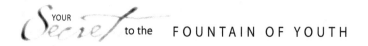

Summary

After less than a few hours of deliberation, the jury reached its innocent verdict following what some Nevada journalists hailed as the "trial of the century" for the state. Although the case never received national publicity, the trial and its outcome have had deep, widespread and lasting ramifications throughout the national medical industry.

Without fear of prosecution, thanks to legal precedence set by this landmark verdict, physicians in both allopathic and alternative medicine practices can continue to issue injectable HGH as an off-label treatment without fear of prosecution so long as they follow acceptable procedures. Meantime, we keep busy telling the public about many clinically proven benefits of this natural hormone.

CHAPTER 2

Discover what "they" don't want you to know

Amazing Nature: Learn how your body makes HGH

Here's the amazing secret that "they" don't want you to know about: An organ called the pituitary gland at the base of your brain generates a natural hormone that creates the characteristics of youth. In both males and females, the body steadily produces this human growth hormone until these levels naturally peak in our mid-20s. From then on, the body's production of vital HGH steadily decreases.

Largely as a result, through their 40s, 50s, 60s and 70s, people exhibit the characteristics of aging. Sex drives decrease, skin wrinkles, brain function deteriorates, body fat increases, the body becomes prone to tiredness and disease, and many other deteriorating characteristics emerge.

A positive, life-changing development started in the mid-1980s when improved technology finally enabled physicians to create injectable HGH in laboratories on a massive scale. This eliminated or severely curtailed the previous method of extracting the substance from cadavers. Laboratory-produced HGH is legal nationwide when prescribed by a licensed physician before being obtained from a licensed pharmacy in the state where the doctor issued the prescription.

Summary

Since childhood, your body naturally produced a hormone that made you useful and strong. Your body's internal creation of this vital substance tapered off beginning from the mid-20s to early 30s, resulting in the characteristics of old age. Yet now, thanks to the advent of technology, you can start receiving this amazing substance again.

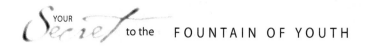

CHAPTER 3

Excited HGH users give positive comments

"HGH has changed my life for the better, in a relatively short period of time," said Jonathan M., a 73-year-old retired casino executive. "For me, the most important benefits were a good increase in energy and what I think is a pretty significant improvement in my ability to recover from strained or sprained muscles. People notice my weight loss most of all, and the change has given them a more positive impression of me."

While every patient displays different characteristics and a unique personality, we list Jonathan as an example of what some patients experience. After conducting the necessary tests to determine if his HGH levels were substandard, we issued him a legal prescription for the hormone shortly after his 72nd birthday. At 5 feet 10 inches tall, during that first visit he weighed 233 pounds, significantly overweight for a man of his age and height.

For the previous eight years Jonathan had been unable to participate in long, quick-paced walks, by far his favorite exercise. Nagging leg cramps and a sharp decrease in energy made him gradually lose interest in walking, until he stopped his daily strolls altogether. His weight problems worsened, gaining an average of five pounds yearly, up from 190 pounds when he stopped walking at age 65.

Today, Jonathan describes himself as happy and vibrant. Following a 51-pound weight loss, at a healthy 182 pounds he enjoys long walks about five times weekly. And when visiting us for regular yearly checkups he always says: "I'm never going to stop taking HGH for as long as I live."

Our HGH patients universally give positive statements about the experience, and none make negative comments of any significance. Some achieve the results they had hoped for, while others say things like, "With all the hype I've heard, I had expected more." Perhaps 10-20 percent of patients voluntarily choose to discontinue their prescriptions. We believe some of those drop-offs occur for financial reasons.

"Everyone keeps telling me how much more attractive I look than before," said Marilyn Z., a 61-year-old receptionist for a major law firm. "I just smile, and never tell them my secret, that this all happened for me thanks to HGH."

Hoping for privacy, Marilyn asked us to avoid revealing her before and after weights, although we're using her as an example and giving a different name for her. With Marilyn's permission, we can report that she had a healthy 35 percent decrease in overall body fat and an 18 percent increase in muscle mass. From Marilyn's perspective and ours as well, the wrinkling on her neck, chin and chest has subsided.

"I want to thank you for this miracle," Veronica B., a 78-year-old housewife told us in her most recent patient visit. When Veronica first came to us a few weeks before her most recent birthday, unsightly age spots riddled her arms, the back of her hands, her face and scattered sections of her neck. Nine months later, following her steady injectable HGH treatments, 95 percent of the markings disappeared.

Veronica's blood tests showed a definite, measurable 35 percent improvement in her hormone levels. In results typical for mature people who use appropriate doses of HGH, we also charted an increase in Veronica's good cholesterol, and a decrease in her bad cholesterol— plus a 15 percent improvement in her heart's ejection fraction, the ability of the heart's left ventricle to pump out blood.

We must be careful to emphasize that there has been no indication whatsoever that injectable HGH can cure, stall or reverse heart disease. As a result, our office never has and never will issue an off-label prescription of HGH as a specific treatment for cardiac problems. Such treatments fall outside our specialty of oncology and alternative

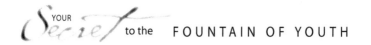

medicine, and no physician should issue such a prescription for this specific type of treatment anyway until more studies are done.

"I never get colds any more," said Dorothy S., an 82-year-old woman who lives in the home of her daughter and son-in-law. "Before getting HGH, during the past seven years or so, it seemed I was always getting colds or the flu."

Dorothy's blood tests concluded that after starting her HGH regimen, the abnormalities in her natural "T" cells improved. With no conclusive evidence to say otherwise, we believe this change improved her body's ability to fight infections.

Lillian S., Dorothy's 78-year-old next-door neighbor who has osteoporosis, visited us after suffering a severe leg break from a fall. Still in a cast during her initial visit, Lillian asked us if we could issue her an HGH prescription to strengthen her bones. We told her, "No," that we never issue off-label prescriptions for such uses, but that a prescription would be possible to improve the HGH levels in her body.

Following the appropriate blood test, we gave Lillian an HGH prescription. Just one month later, she told us that her fracture had healed twice faster than her family doctor had told her to expect. Our tests showed that her bone density increased within 12 months.

Smiling, Lillian told us, "There has been another change that I hadn't anticipated. Everyone in my family is amazed because my mind definitely is much sharper than before."

Three months after beginning her HGH treatments began, for the first time in years Lillian started playing board games like checkers, and she began watching the TV game show "Jeopardy" with her grandchildren—occasionally belting out correct answers before some of the brightest contestants. Before taking HGH, Lillian never came close to displaying such sharpness.

Until more conclusive studies are complete, we would never consider injectable HGH as a treatment to prevent or delay the onset of dementia. Yet we're pleased to report regular and consistent results on mental acuity such as those enjoyed by Lillian.

Every week or so, we hear positive comments from HGH patients who say they're amazed. Byron B., a 67-year-old patient, always refers to his prescription as "The Fountain of Youth that no one else knows about." While more intensive studies are needed to make such a claim, we agree with Byron—at least in the sense that most people remain unaware of legal HGH and our clinical results consistently give positive findings.

Summary

Growing numbers of mature people nationwide are providing positive comments about their results with HGH when administered under proper medical supervision, although you never hear of these extraordinary testimonies in the mainstream media.

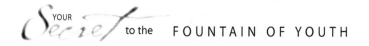
CHAPTER 4

Average HGH results inspire mature people

Many of us often hear the buzz-phrase "there's no such thing as average." Even so, based on our laboratory results and comments from patients, we're able to give a brief description of changes that occur in a typical 70-year-old woman who starts taking injectable HGH on a regular basis, as prescribed by a certified physician.

By this stage in life, this woman—whom we'll call Alice—has slowed down considerably in all physical activities. Like clockwork, she retires to bed at 9 o'clock sharp each night, a few hours earlier than her pattern from a few decades earlier. Heavyset with large bags under her eyes, Alice usually awakens by 6 o'clock in the morning but feels tired through much of the day.

Retired like her husband, Fred, she handles their grocery shopping but always feels dead tired by the time she gets home. Alice's decreasing strength, endurance and agility have forced her into a predictable routine.

We know that proclaiming Alice as "typical" is politically incorrect and unfair, since many 70-year-old women feel far more vibrant than she—while others show even less energy. Yet from our experience, her physical attributes are far from atypical.

In a nutshell, Alice had gotten "old" at least when compared to many women her age and especially when compared to young adults. While many people scoff at the mere mention of the word "old," that's how she was perceived by much of society and even by herself.

Enjoy shining results

At age 71, one year after beginning an injectable HGH regimen, Alice glowed with confidence. People who had not seen her for several years instantly proclaimed how much better she looks and seems, and she openly admits that, "You're right."

You see, by this point—slimmer than before—Alice occasionally stayed up late watching TV, or going out to the theater with her husband. Once they get home, she enjoys intimate time with Fred.

Unlike just a year ago, Alice often extends her grocery shopping trips by taking leisurely strolls through their community's largest shopping mall—sometimes to buy lingerie or luxurious evening gowns. For the first time in a decade, she arranged a two-week ocean cruise for two, surprising her husband.

Before taking HGH, Alice occasionally became frustrated at her frequent inability to open something as mundane as a pickle jar. Back then, she had no choice other than to ask Fred to help with such simple chores. Today marks a far different atmosphere. Alice's improved muscle mass enables her to open such containers herself with ease.

Around six months after Alice started taking prescribed HGH, Fred began noticing that she smiled much more frequently than before. This devoted husband realized that his wife had found a new sense of happiness. Should the credit go to HGH? All Fred knew for sure was that she looked better than ever, and their relationship had improved.

Who is a macho-macho man?

During Alice's first six months of taking HGH, Fred balked at her continual suggestions that he try the hormone. Initially, pride prevented him from showing much curiosity, at least openly. Finally, struck by a sense of mystery, one morning Fred snuck to the same physician's office that Alice had been visiting.

Fred went through the necessary blood test to determine whether his natural HGH levels had decreased below those of average young adults.

As soon as Doctor Pickering told him that "your HGH levels are low," Fred asked for and got a prescription for a one-month supply.

At first, Fred gave these injections little thought, administering the hormones when alone in the bathroom late at night so that Alice wouldn't know. During those first few weeks, Fred went about his typical daily routine, which pretty much meant staying home glued to the TV. At age 75 he had little energy or motivation.

Then, a few weeks after beginning his HGH regimen, Fred began bounding into the kitchen for snacks. Re-energized, he finally confessed to Alice that he had been taking the hormone.

"I've noticed this positive change in you the past several days," Alice told her husband.

Blessed with new-found zest, at Alice's insistence, a week later Fred made his first trip to the golf course in a decade. When in his mid-60s, this retired civil engineer had stopped participating in this, his favorite sport, due to nagging aches and pains. By that point his aging body usually took weeks or months—if at all—to recover from these bothersome discomforts.

This time, just a few months after his 75th birthday, Fred enjoyed a full round of golf while suffering only minor discomfort in his left shoulder. A single aspirin made the pain go away, and since then he has had a blast in weekly excursions to his favorite links. As an added benefit, during the months that followed Fred developed solid friendships with new-found golfing buddies.

Genders from different planets

Alice and Fred serve as an ideal couple when learning the different reactions between genders. At age 70, Alice began her HGH regimen but it took a full year until her muscles had improved enough to open pickle jars herself. Meantime, her libido took awhile to click into higher gear.

By contrast, shortly after Fred began receiving regular HGH injections at age 75, the benefits he received were almost immediate and much more diverse than hers. This man's increase in energy enabled him to resume an old favorite sport, while Alice previously had no such favorite activity.

His forays to the golf course proved more vigorous and intense than Alice's new but occasional leisurely strolls through the shopping mall.

While each benefited, they individually would have given vastly different in-person interviews on how HGH impacted their lives. Despite their different results, Alice and Fred each became dedicated to using HGH—but for contrasting reasons.

Summary

While results vary among individual patients, a vast majority of mature people who take injectable HGH report significant health improvements, and our clinical results consistently back up their positive reactions.

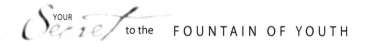

CHAPTER 5

Suddenly: "It's more cool than ever to be old"

Many of today's youngest boomers fondly recall a popular tune by Huey Lewis and the News, lyrics proclaiming that "It's hip to be square." With the advent of HGH, many of these same people could soon seek to change the lyrics to "It's cool to be old."

Thanks to the increasing popularity of injectable HGH, those who can afford the hormone and who choose to get such treatments exhibit greater zest and desire for life while gaining respect from our youth.

At present, we're unaware of any formal society or association dedicated solely to seniors who use this hormone. Of course, numerous organizations advocate the rights of seniors, including the American Association of Retired Persons or AARP.

The worldwide, 25,000-member American Academy of Anti-Aging Medicine advocates prescribed HGH, in cases where a medical professional deems such treatment as appropriate. The power of the international news media should help increase the popularity of HGH in other countries as our government's conspiracy becomes known.

Discover the benefits

Once people decide to seek a prescription for injectable HGH, many begin to realize the significance of this life-changing decision. Although many of our patients have heard of great features the substance provides, they sometimes get overly excited without first keeping the treatment's many benefits in perspective.

Determined to give them a clear understanding of what likely will happen, on occasion we explain to individual patients the results of

HGH chronicled on a variety of characteristics in the human body. Many seniors visiting our clinic for the first time get motivated when discovering the point-by-point detailed descriptions that soon will follow.

To put this into clear perspective, we first explain how basic functions of the human body operate in healthy young individuals up to age 25. These many features include skin texture, heart efficiency, sexual desire, cholesterol levels, muscle mass, body fat, overall organ function, and energy levels—plus a variety of other bodily functions.

Then, for each individual aspect of our body's pertinent operations, our clinic can list how overall healthiness deteriorates as natural HGH production diminishes. From here, we describe how the injectable version of this hormone is likely to help or reverse everything from deteriorating eyesight to problems with flexibility—if at all.

Summary

The number of mature people who are able to afford injectable bio-identical human growth hormone will increase markedly during the next several years, as more people discover the many health benefits that "they" don't want you to know.

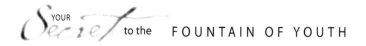

CHAPTER 6

Our clinical results give irrefutable proof

The so-called "powers that be" don't want you to know the irrefutable, clinically proven results. Thanks largely to our own extensive research we're able to show point-by-point data on numerous vital physical characteristics.

The conspirators who sought my arrest and conviction are trying hard to keep you from learning the proven medical data on HGH that you're about to discover. If they had their way, at this very moment, medical professionals like us would be rotting in jail in order to keep you from knowing the truth.

Huge pharmaceutical companies collectively and individually generate billions of dollars by selling expensive drugs. Many of these pharmaceuticals treat mature-age-related symptoms such as hypertension, high cholesterol, age spots and osteoporosis—all symptoms that legally prescribed HGH can reverse, curtail or eliminate at much lower expense.

Since our bodies naturally produce HGH, the substance is tolerated and effective in mature people when administered in appropriate doses. From our view, high-paid pharmaceutical company lobbyists cringe at the thought that here you're able to learn the truth.

Our clinic has chronicled many dozens of positive results provided by HGH, on everything from the skin and liver function, to bone density and body fat. In each instance, we have carefully and scientifically listed the benefits of naturally produced HGH for people from youth though the young adult years.

The clinic also chronicles what happens to our bodies during the aging process from our mid-20s through maturity. Using what happens naturally with HGH during the growth and aging process as a benchmark, we're able to specifically list what benefits—if any—that injectable HGH provides for mature people. Among our many point-by-point findings on specific areas or functions of the body:

The Skin

- **Youth through young adult:** Often called the body's largest organ, the skin protects people from outside invaders while performing many vital functions that include sweat glands for heating and cooling, plus the vital senses of touch. Healthy skin keeps essential fluids within the body while shielding or protecting other organs. Except for acne during the teens and young adult period, the skin of most young people is relatively blemish-free and wrinkle-free.

- **Mid-20s through maturity:** The skin gradually begins to wrinkle, and then more progressively as time passes from the 40s and beyond. The incidence of cancerous or unsightly moles or lesions increases markedly. Age spots, commonly referred to as liver spots, begin appearing on the back of the hands, neck, face and other regions.

- **Upon getting HGH during maturity:** Many wrinkles diminish somewhat or disappear altogether. Most or all liver spots disappear. Clinical results remain inconclusive on how much—if at all—the advent of HGH reduces the incidence of skin cancers. We think injectable HGH lessens the likelihood of such diseases, but more studies are needed to prove that.

The Libido

- **Youth through young adult:** In healthy individuals, the libido increases in intensity as the years progress, particularly past puberty. People's desire for physical intimacy peaks during the late teens through the mid-20s.

- **Mid-20s through maturity:** People gradually have less desire for physical contact. The libido's intensity steadily wanes, to the point where many women during menopause never think of sex. Many men begin feeling less passionate. Despite the advent of erectile dysfunction drugs such as Viagra®, large percentage of men become unwilling or physically unable to pursue sexual intercourse.

- **Upon getting HGH during maturity:** Both genders report increases in sexual desire, particularly men. Although, overall, women report less of an increase in libido, mano experience an increase in desire.

Energy Levels

- **Youth through young adult:** Healthy people possess increasingly boundless energy, in some instances even when eating little or no food for limited periods. Some children play so much they lose any sense of time. College students and young adults are legendary for going days at a time with just a few hours of nightly sleep.

- **Mid-20s through maturity:** Energy levels decrease slowly through the early 30s, before dropping off at a steadily increasing rate from the early 40s and beyond. For some seniors, exercise and restricting foods to low-calorie, high-protein meals can boost energy somewhat. But most people experience a sharp decrease in vitality, especially during their 60s and 70s. Many have difficulty exercising due to physical challenges caused by aging.

- **Upon getting HGH during maturity:** Many—but not all— patients report a significant increase in vigor. Some resume games or sports they had once dropped such as golf. Others begin low-intensity exercise like walking. Overall, men report a greater increase in energy than women. Most females become more vibrant as well.

The Bones

- **Youth through young adult:** Beginning from childbirth, the bones grow until emerging as our mature primary adult lifetime physical frames in the early 20s. Thanks to natural HGH, during this 25-year period most bone fractures heal fast—sometimes amazingly so. The bone marrow also plays the essential role of creating blood-forming precursors for red blood cells, white blood cells and platelets.

- **Mid-20s through maturity:** Due to the aging process coupled with decreasing HGH, bone density steadily decreases, greatly increasing the probability of fractures among people 60 and older. Particularly in women, severe cases of osteoporosis make the bones appear as if hole-ridden Swiss cheese. Hip fractures are a leading cause of death among mature females; most women who suffer hip fractures die of other related complications within a few years.

- **Upon getting HGH in maturity:** On a consistent basis, for both men and women bone density increases, sometimes up to 1 percent per year. This decreases the likelihood of severe fractures, a significant development, especially among women.

The Heart's Efficiency

- **Youth through young adult:** In healthy individuals, with each beat the heart's left ventricle pumps out most blood into the aorta, thereby increasing the likelihood of good overall cardiovascular health. Physicians use the term "ejection fraction" when measuring this degree of efficiency. Most healthy people from their teens through early 20s have an ejection fraction level greater than 55 percent of blood that had been in the heart.

- **Mid-20s through maturity:** Partly due to a decrease in the body's production of HGH, ejection fraction levels begin to decrease as the heart muscle's efficiency decreases. In some individuals, this change emerges as a primary or secondary factor leading to heart disease, fatal in some instances. For the most part, people with ejection fractions of less than 50 percent are considered to have heart disease and may have congestive heart failure.

- **Upon getting HGH in maturity:** Among healthy individuals whose hearts have not yet been irreversibly damaged, patients experience a marked improvement in their ejection fraction. This, in turn, can result in overall improvements in health throughout the body. However, to this point medical professionals have yet to complete comprehensive research, partly due to restrictions the federal government imposes on the use of HGH in the general population—other than in cases where physicians issue "off-label" prescriptions.

Memory

- **Youth through young adult:** Healthy young children have remarkable memories, particularly as they learn languages and other vital skills. Teens and young adults sometimes hone their memories, often capable of answering basic queries almost from the millisecond that they hear a question. These cognitive abilities also help them respond fast to sudden dangerous situations, such as while driving a car that goes out of control—using their brains to make vital instant decisions.

- **Mid-20s through maturity:** The brain responds to emergency situations much slower than during youth. Mature people react slower to life-threatening situations, such as slamming the brakes when it's too late—while young people lack such problems in some similar situations. Also, the memory fades, and people gradually lose cognitive skills they once took for granted. Beginning in their 40s, many people start forgetting phone numbers they once knew in a flash, or they lose car keys or other possessions with greater frequency. Even people who lack early signs of Alzheimer's disease sometimes walk into rooms, only to suddenly forget why they went there.

- **Upon getting HGH during maturity:** Our clinical results show that these people enjoy an increase in mental acuity and sharpness, while experiencing a greater overall interest in life. These changes make them feel better about themselves, and many even feel like learning again. Yet more studies are needed. For now, we think injectable HGH may delay or eliminate the onset of dementia.

Eyesight and Hearing

- **Youth through young adult:** For most children and young adults, eyesight is keen at around 20/20 vision, while many can hear pins drop from long distances. Of course, plenty of children need corrective eyewear or hearing aids, but a vast majority of them lack such problems.

- **Mid-20s through maturity:** The overall quality of eyesight and hearing decreases. For the first time in the late 20s through 40s, many people get their first eyeglasses or contact lenses. A small percentage of people discover that they need hearing aids.

- **Upon getting HGH during maturity:** Again, partly as a result of restrictions imposed by the federal government on the ability of physicians to issue "off-label" prescriptions for HGH, we lack any conclusions or opinions on whether this hormone decreases the incidence of cataracts, glaucoma or retinal detachments, or if it improves hearing. Even so, we believe injectable HGH strengthens eye muscles, reducing certain vision problems while also decreasing the need for reading glasses.

Cholesterol

• **Youth through young adult:** For the most part, in healthy individuals the body regulates the levels of HDL, commonly known as good cholesterol, and LDL, the bad cholesterol that can lead to heart problems or coronary artery disease. By contrast, HDL works to diminish harmful triglycerides, thereby making arteries healthier.

• **Mid-20s through maturity:** As the aging process progresses, the vascular systems of most people begin to deteriorate. The body's control of HDL and LDL levels gets off kilter, increasing the incidence of coronary disease. Life-debilitating or fatal afflictions emerge, including the clogging of arteries.

• **Upon getting HGH during maturity:** On a consistent basis, the lipid profiles that we take on these patients show improvement in their levels of HDL and LDL. We never have prescribed HGH as a treatment for cholesterol problems. Yet we've discovered these improvements as a positive, consistent side effect when issuing "off-label" prescriptions of HGH for anti-aging treatments.

The muscles

• **Youth through young adult:** The muscles enable us to move, while defining our bodies so that we can attract the opposite gender as young adults, and to perform vital activities such as physical labor. Sturdy muscles enable healthy people to keep their balance, often providing flexibility and strength. The muscles serve as significant tools for young people as they suffer falls or attacks, in some cases enabling them to avoid or ward off potential injury.

- **Mid-20s through maturity:** The muscles lose their previous size and strength as natural levels of HGH decrease. Mature people in their 60s and 70s sometimes lack enough strength to keep their balance, increasing the incidence of accidental falls. Since the muscles and tendons also play a key role in maintaining healthy joints, some people begin suffering problems in these areas.

- **Upon getting HGH during maturity:** On a consistent basis, muscles throughout the body increase in size and strength. In the vast majority of individuals, we track growth in biceps, triceps, calf muscles, quadriceps, and the neck muscles. Many joint problems decrease or disappear. And people find they're able to resume strenuous activities. Men, particularly, consider this benefit as significant as they resume favorite sporting activities ranging from golf, tennis and bicycling to walking. Some women report similar results.

Body fat

- **Youth through young adult:** Even during infancy, childhood, puberty and the young adult stage, we all need healthy amounts of body fat—primarily to store energy. Young people who eat too much food often gain excessive weight, sometimes becoming obese. For the most part a majority of healthy young people find it relatively easy to lose weight fast, and some never gain excess pounds at all thanks largely to their naturally high energy levels.

- **Mid-20s through maturity:** Progressively as the years pass, the body has less energy, burning off increasingly smaller percentages of fat. Calorie-restriction and exercise become less efficient during the 30s and 40s. Losing weight becomes increasingly difficult for people older than 50. Occasional weight loss becomes short-term as low energy levels persist.

- **Upon getting HGH during maturity:** An increase in energy levels, coupled with larger muscle mass, burns off calories and decreases the body's overall percentage of fat. This makes the person look more attractive, while increasing the ability to move about and expend energy. Our clinical results regularly and consistently show decreases in body fat.

Hip-to-waist ratio

- **Youth through young adult:** Especially during the late teens and young adult period, an excellent hip-to-waist ratio is often considered a sign of attractiveness. Even more important, many physicians view a good ratio as a sign of superior overall health— less prone to diseases such as diabetes or prostate cancer. Waists usually are smaller than hips or posterior areas. Young women have a greater hip-to-waist ratio than men in order to endure the birthing process.

- **Mid-20s through maturity:** The sizes of bellies and posteriors often increase, outside the range of ideal ratios. The advent of disease rises, while people become less physically attractive.

- **Upon getting HGH during maturity:** Hip-to-waist ratios improve thanks to the increase in muscle mass and the overall decrease in body fat. This makes mature people who take HGH appear more attractive. Yet for now, we lack studies on whether this improved hip-to-waist ratio correlates to any decrease in disease.

Healing ability

- **Youth through young adult:** Healthy individuals heal amazingly fast, largely because HGH levels are surging through their bodies. The growth factor often enables them to recover within days or mere weeks. Young people injured in car accidents or wounded in combat often fully recover from trauma that could have easily killed a much older person.

- **Mid-20s through maturity:** People from their mid-30s and beyond heal much slower from severe wounds, thereby increasing the probability of extreme or fatal infections. Also, those recovering from surgeries tend to heal much slower than young people who receive the same operations.

- **Upon getting HGH during maturity:** We're unaware of any formal studies on what impact HGH has on the abilities of mature people to heal. However, some patients tell us they recover much faster from sports injuries such as muscle strains. Comprehensive studies are necessary before we can reach a definitive conclusion.

Immunity

- **Youth through young adult:** In healthy individuals, the body creates white blood cells to ward off infections. Various white cell types each employ "T" cell receptors that fight invaders and help eliminate infections. At times, invading viruses such as the flu, measles or the common cold cause adverse symptoms ranging from fever to sore throats and runny noses. Most of the time the immunity system prevents or destroys the worst symptoms, with recovery relatively fast, usually within a matter of days.

- **Mid-20s through maturity:** Due to the natural decrease in HGH, the immune system becomes less efficient. Abnormalities appear in the blood's anti-infection "B" cells and "T" cells, resulting in increased infections. During outbreaks of severe flu, authorities warn that the worst symptoms often target mature people. Infections including pneumonia are among leading causes of death among seniors.

- **Upon getting HGH during maturity:** On a consistent basis, we see a decrease in abnormalities in the vital anti-infection B cells and T cells. Although there have been no studies on whether these improvements decrease the probability of infections, we believe that's the case. Comprehensive research is still needed.

Overall organ function

- **Youth through young adult:** An extremely small percentage of children suffer from problems with vital organs such as the heart, kidneys and pancreas. Thanks largely to HGH naturally produced within the body, organs grow to their mature size during this stage.

- **Mid-20s through maturity:** Decreased HGH output can contribute to the advent of heart disease. Yet, barring this, as an overall group, in most people the internal organs continue to function well enough to keep a person alive—until inevitable and eventual death. Even in people as old as 90, unless they already suffer from such maladies as heart or kidney problems, for the most part the organs function fine up to the end of life.

- **Upon getting HGH during maturity:** Other than chronicled improvements in cardiac function, we've found no evidence that HGH improves the organs individually and as an overall group—although it's likely the hormone contributes to healthy organ function.

Life expectancy

- **Youth through young adult:** A person born in the United States today could expect to live about 77-81 years.

- **Mid-20s through maturity:** Barring the advent of cataclysmic events such as war, famine or the onset of new horrific diseases, the average person born in the U.S. in 2009 should expect to live to about 2086-2090.

- **Upon getting HGH during maturity:** We lack any hard clinical evidence to indicate that mature people who use injectable HGH live longer than should otherwise be expected. Yet we think they will live at least somewhat longer, and our studies clearly show that the overall quality of their lives improves while taking HGH. Even so, the proverbial jury is still out on this, and far more research is necessary.

Summary

Our irrefutable laboratory results, coupled with universally positive comments from mature HGH users nationwide, prove that the government, Big Pharma and standard-medicine physicians are flat-out wrong when they claim the human growth hormone is useless or dangerous when prescribed in recommended doses. Thousands of articles in both the allopathic and alternative literature support these findings.

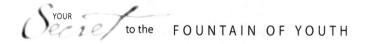

CHAPTER 7

HGH will attract many of the nearly 80 million baby boomers

As word spreads about the many amazing benefits of legal injectable HGH, we foresee a huge increase in the use of this substance by the Baby Boom Generation as it emerges into retirement years and beyond.

By some estimates, many of the whopping 78.2 million people born between 1946 and 1964 will seek any legal means possible to maintain their youthfulness or vitality.

During their 40s and 50s, many of the oldest Boomers started hopping onto the get-youthful bandwagon. From the late '80s to the present, swarms of these middle-aged people bought Jane Fonda's aerobic videos and Jack LaLanne® exercise equipment.

Suddenly good-health enthusiasts, these people took up jogging while running through a maze of diets including the Atkins Diet®, the ZoneDiet®, South Beach® and more. Along the way, lots of Boomers saw their parents wasting away in nursing homes.

Eager to avoid entering such demeaning human warehouses themselves, huge numbers of these individuals will flock to legal injectable HGH. Many of our patients proclaim eagerness to seize this technology, gaining vitality and improving brain function.

Lots of people older than 50 who use injectable HGH wake up early in the morning feeling rejuvenated, often after staying up late the previous night to dance, watch television, enjoy physical intimacy, or other activities.

Many also enjoy playing games that require mental sharpness, everything from chess to poker, or even watching the popular TV game show "Jeopardy," sometimes giving answers before contestants.

An added blessing comes to those unlucky enough to suffer everything from minor or more serious injuries, surgical wounds and wounds from serious falls. Injectable HGH enables mature people to recover much faster than before taking this natural substance, while the chances of serious or debilitating injury actually decrease thanks to HGH. Our studies show that bone density often increases by several percent after a few years of taking HGH, in some cases eliminating osteoporosis.

What about regaining a youthful appearance?

None of our HGH patients who are age 50 or older look 25 years old. Nonetheless, a high percentage of these individuals look or feel 10 or 15 years younger than their actual age.

Some significant changes occur in the look, feel and texture of the skin, which becomes thicker—making these patients have a less weathered or wrinkled appearance.

Prior to taking injectable HGH, just about everyone over age 50 has what the general public commonly refers to as "age spots" or "liver spots," often on the back of their hands together with ugly blemishes. These usually disappear after taking human growth hormone.

In what has become an everyday process that generates little surprise, many of these patients regain a degree of elasticity in their skin. Much of the time, this makes the tone or constitution of the face, neck and arms appear tighter and firmer.

Because HGH improves liver function and the body's ability to ward off toxins, in some cases unsightly moles or warts fade or disappear.

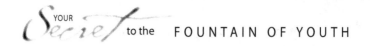

These changes give an impression of youthfulness, since such blemishes are associated with the stigma of old age.

Enjoy a glowing aura

Have you ever bumped into someone after being away from them for awhile, only to find they seemed more vibrant, youthful and happier than before? Perhaps they've had a well-done facelift or recovered psychologically from a death in the family, a divorce or a job loss. Your instinctive reaction motivates you to tell them that they look fantastic.

Lots of our patients who use injectable HGH report similar reactions. Surprised and smiling acquaintances might say: "Holy cow, you've changed for the better. Did you retire wealthy or something?"

These patients enjoy greater vitality, a zestful energy they lacked before. This change, in turn, often enables older patients to get more exercise, engaging in activities as simple as strolls in shopping malls.

Increases in exercise can improve organ function, especially the heart. Think of this as a double bonus. Our tests consistently show that HGH improves cardiac function, even among patients who decide to get little or no additional exercise.

The improved heart function, in turn, re-energizes the flow of vital blood and oxygen to the brain. As a result, many HGH patients become joyful when their memories improve, they answer questions faster, and they start engaging in lively conversations. Patients with positive mental attitudes and better brain function enjoy greater happiness and an improved overall quality of life.

Better brain function that results from the use of injectable HGH often leads to sharp improvements in the ability to make decisions. And boosted by higher energy levels, these patients often choose or engage in life-fulfilling activities.

Mature people who resume or start such interests often find a glow, energy and pizzazz that had been missing from their lives. For many, these changes result in a new "meaning" or "purpose" for life—igniting the will to live.

Improved exercise tolerance

Most children heal extremely fast from minor cuts, scrapes, sprains and even bone fractures, while mature people lack or have little such natural healing power. For the young, most of these seemingly miraculous recoveries result from large quantities of human growth hormones that their bodies generate.

To the delight of many seniors, our clinical results indicate that recovery rates from injuries increase markedly among mature people who use injectable HGH. A large percentage also tell us they suffer fewer aches after minor sports activities.

Before taking HGH, many who tried to resume these activities made a sharp cutback in such exercise or quit altogether. Mysterious aches, strains and sprains became too much to tolerate.

Mature women using human growth hormones could rarely be mistaken for bathing beauties in Miss America contests. Also, we'll never try to convince older men that by merely taking HGH they'll soon end up looking like Charles Atlas strolling down Muscle Beach.

Yet our studies regularly and consistently show that over a period of time mature people who use injectable HGH grow in overall muscle structure.

Just as in nature during their young-adult years, an increase in muscle mass for seniors also generates a decrease in body fat. Love handles around the waist decrease in size or disappear.

On occasion, posteriors shrink, while the thighs and neckline also tend to firm up somewhat. Such structural changes can make the person look more alluring, not to mention being far more attractive. Just as important, non-fatty increases in structural mass connote overall good health. Many patients proclaim, "I feel better than ever."

From hundreds of years ago when the Greeks launched the first Olympic-style games, through the 20th Century to the present day, physical training experts have stressed the need for athletes to excel in three categories—strength, agility and endurance.

When compared to those in the senior population, teenagers and young adults reign as far superior in these physical skills. As the decades pass, mature people lose much of their strength and their ability to move about at ease freely with little or no pain. Many seniors get tired often as their endurance fades.

Now, the good news is spreading that injectable HGH can stall or reverse these natural trends to varying degrees in each individual. The results we've chronicled remain undeniably positive.

Lights, cameras, action!

Motivated by stories such as those of Alice and Fred, everyone from middle-class families to some movie stars has contacted our office for advice on how they can get this natural substance. People travel from around the country to visit us, though in many instances they could get such prescriptions in their own communities.

Some of the world's most popular action movie stars visit our office, where we give these men and women the appropriate tests, before possibly issuing them legitimate prescriptions for injectable HGH. Average citizens just like you hold the same rights involving the use of prescribed human growth hormone.

What should you tell people?

Some patients find themselves so absorbed with getting their first HGH prescriptions that they initially put little thought, if any, into what to tell people they know.

One logical answer dictates a keep-quiet strategy, since some people—especially those prone to jealousy—might pepper you with a continual maze of unwanted or bothersome questions. Pesky queries could spring forth, ranging from "Do you really think you look better?" to "Don't you think this apparent change is only psychological?"

These questions, in turn, might tend to make you think or ponder more than necessary about the benefits. Could you end up asking yourself, "Am I really getting a lot friskier than just a few months ago, and do I really have a lot more energy—or is all this merely a placebo effect, something that's strictly in my head?"

We tell patients to let results speak for themselves. And on the question of what to tell people, consider:

- **Keep Quiet:** This often remains the best tactic. What people never know for sure lacks the potential to bother them.

- **Limited info:** Tell only a handful of people, heightening a sense of urgency by giving only sketchy details.

- **Openness:** Make this quest a tell-all journey, chronicling for your acquaintances as many details as you want, from changes in your blood results to the disappearance of age spots.

The gender trap

As a group using injectable HGH, men enjoy faster results than women in getting their desired changes. Within two to four weeks of starting their regimens, large numbers of men say their libidos are already re-energizing and they feel much more energy. Overall by this early stage, women tell us their results are far less pronounced.

So far, we have yet to pinpoint a specific reason why the changes seem more dramatic in men. Our initial theory tells us that perhaps injectable HGH synergizes better or faster with male hormones than with female estrogen profiles.

Men often tell us that they feel so much better shortly after starting these prescriptions that "I never want to get off of it." Conversely, in some cases, although women proclaim that they feel better, some of them do not seem as impressed with the changes. So, a small percentage of women lack motivation to continue.

Experts in the body's natural hormones, endocrinologists, have been unable to give us a definitive reason. Perhaps an answer rests in the fact that, psychologically, many males seem more motivated to exercise than females. While there certainly are exceptions between the genders, as separate overall groups this might hold true.

Taking these concerns a step further, maybe the increase in energy levels afforded by injectable HGH motivates men to move their bodies more than the substance does to women—resulting in an overall sense of improvement among males. Certainly, more studies should continue.

Interesting result comparisons

While specific practices vary among people, countries and cultures, overall the male is usually the aggressor when instigating and eventually while having physical relations with females. Thus, men might sense a greater benefit from HGH than women in this regard, since men have more to gain—at least sexually—from the increased energy that this hormone provides.

Injectable HGH might naturally produce more muscle mass in mature males than the same hormone produces in older females. In addition, women's bodies generally have less of a need for the many benefits that human growth hormones generate. In nature, men have—and need—more musculature than women.

Many women like HGH because the hormone increases their strength. The substance gives females a measurable increase in bone density, a change that—as already noted—actually could prevent death. A large percentage of older females suffer falls, and women who break their hips often die within a few years of sustaining such fractures.

Adding spice to the mix, women also like the fact that as an overall group, their cardiac function improves thanks to HGH. This helps improve the quality of their lives, while also possibly increasing their life spans.

Summary

As increasing numbers of people use injectable HGH, we're continually learning about more positive benefits never previously known. The research on the benefits of HGH replacement in the aging population is certain to reveal amazing results as studies mature.

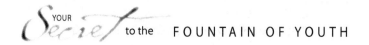

CHAPTER 8

The Eternal Question: What causes old age?

Baby Boomers and the generation that preceded them were often told early in life that "old people" are either laughable or bothersome. During the '40s, '50s and '60s, society seemed to forget the fact that someday many of that era's youngsters would reach maturity.

In "Rowan and Martin's Laugh-In," a hit TV series from 1967 to 1973, many of the biggest laughs came when mature guys got portrayed as nothing but comic dirty old men. Like children, senior citizens were supposed to "be seen and not heard."

Even today as overall life spans increase, our culture imposes a mindset that the traits of growing old are the equivalent of a disease that should be removed. People over age 50 rush to get liposuctions, tummy tucks, breast implants, face lifts, hair implants, eyebrow lifts, nose reconstruction, Botox® cosmetic injections, facial fillers and more—all terms absent from the overall public mindset as recently as the mid-1960s.

Along the way, perhaps you have given little or no thought as to why or how people age, or even what biological mechanisms make us youthful, vibrant and pleasant to look at until we pass into the older adult stage. Gaining a keen understanding of these basic biological mechanisms goes a long way in developing valuable knowledge of the many benefits and uses of injectable HGH.

Your biological clock keeps ticking

From the beginnings of recorded history, humans have grappled with the mystery of why people age. In the Book of Genesis, the earliest chronicles from the Holy Bible, Adam and Eve enjoyed vitality until they eventually aged and died—punishment for imbibing in forbidden fruit.

On a scientific level, Aristotle, the famed Greek philosopher and teacher who lived from 384-322 B.C., studied, indexed and discussed the life spans of various species. Galen, an ancient Greek physician, contributed to the subject by writing extensively on the mystery of aging during the second and third centuries after the birth of Christ.

In "The History of Life and Death," English philosopher, statesmen and essayist Sir Francis Bacon, who lived from 1561 to 1626, claimed that "men of old age object too much, consult too long, adventure too little, repent too soon, seldom drive business home to the full period—but they content themselves with mediocrity of success."

The legendary playwright William Shakespeare, 1564-1616, described old age as "second childishness and mere oblivion, sans teeth, sans eyes, sans taste, sans everything"—adding that old people "have a plentiful lack of wit."

This leads us to wonder whether Shakespeare would have taken injectable HGH in the final years prior to his mysterious death at the tender age of 52. To this day, historians argue about the direct cause of Shakespeare's demise, with theories ranging from cerebral hemorrhage to a sudden cardiac arrest.

As our clinical results show, injectable HGH improves cardiac function and the overall health of other vital organs, perhaps decreasing the likelihood of such fatal afflictions. If given a choice, Shakespeare undoubtedly would have queried, "To take HGH or not take HGH? That is the question."

Today, disagreement reigns supreme

Today, medical professionals seem to grapple with more theories on the cause of aging than there were gladiators at the Coliseum in Rome.

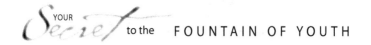

Sure enough, in the modern arena of public opinion, seen everywhere from the Internet to flash-in-the-pan publications sold in bookstores, conflicting theories abound on the supposed causes and "cures" for aging.

Long before the current forms of electronic media emerged, in the early 1900s Russian microbiologist Ilya Ilyich Mechnikov conducted pioneering research on the immune system. In 1908, he won the Nobel Prize in Medicine for a groundbreaking study on cells, the immune system and the study of aging.

Known in the West as Elie Metchnikoff, he developed a theory concluding that aging was caused "by a build-up of toxins from the intestinal tract, which over a period of a life span contributed to aging and ultimately death."

Like invading microbes, during the ensuing century other scientists, physicians and homeopaths developed a maze of vastly different theories. From our view, the actual biological factors that cause aging might involve a handful or even a large number of these conclusions.

A sparkling new term emerges: "Oldie-Boomer"

In a sense, Baby Boomers are steadily evolving into what we might call "Oldie-Boomers." Every 30 seconds another person in our country—born from 1945 through 1964—reaches the milestone half-century mark.

Back in the 1960s, TV ads for the heartburn and indigestion-relief medicine Alka-Seltzer® saturated the airwaves with the catchy tune, "Oh, what a relief it is!" People everywhere wanted a quick-fix for a wide variety of health problems. If we could put a man on the moon, why couldn't experts cure the common cold, and old age for that matter?

To understand why finding a cure has continued to boggle the minds of physicians, we need an insight into why humans progressively show the characteristics of old age and eventually die. By some accounts, Mother Nature has programmed each person with an internal biological clock that tells our cells when to wind down and cease functioning.

You might call this a nature-mandated Planned Obsolescence for Humans, like cars built by auto manufacturers so that they'll break down after a certain number of miles. In humans, physicians have pinpointed a program that sets pre-designated times when milestone events occur.

Medical professionals and just about every parent knows the ranges in time after birth that infants will get those first teeth, crawl, walk, learn initial words, and start talking in cohesive sentences. Growth spurts and sexual maturity evolve during puberty. Within a few short decades, the degenerative phase cruelly starts to kick into gear.

Compounding the problem, current theories of aging on the cellular molecular level say that besides the pre-set clock, we also age due to a random series of adverse events. Under this realm of thinking, each individual sits within a designated slot on a proverbial roulette wheel. Whether the odds are in your favor or not, if the "ball" of fate lands in your slot, it's time to start aging faster than your peers of the same age.

That dreaded series of random adverse events

Perhaps you've known people who aged rapidly after sudden severe injury or the rapid onset of illness. We believe many of these individuals, including some of our favorite celebrities, could have been helped by injectable HGH.

Without getting into too much integral medical jargon, when considering such tragedies, you might want to know that in scientific terms the random theories of aging rely on chance—coupled with the notion that organisms get older because of a random series of events. Wear and tear on one vital organ might cause a domino effect, sparking a series of organ failures as aging accelerates faster than nature originally intended.

The random theories with the greatest validity involve the "wear-and-tear theory" and the "neuroendocrine theory," a scientific term for the body's complicated system of bio-chemicals that govern the release of hormones to the organs.

When we're young, the neuroendocrine system enables hormones to regulate vital body functions, everything from reactions to stress and sexual activity to determining the individual's ultimate height, weight and organ growth.

But in the neuroendocrine theory, these systems malfunction as we age. During our mature years, the hypothalamus, within the brain above the pituitary gland, starts to regulate the release of various hormones without the great efficiency that it once achieved during youth. Thus, the signs of aging emerge.

Consider environmental factors

The environment where an individual lives also plays an integral role. Survivors of the World War II nuclear bombings of Hiroshima and Nagasaki, and the Three Mile Island and Chernobyl nuclear reactor disasters suffered a much higher rate of cancers than people outside their regions. Individuals within these danger zones aged and died faster than average.

People living in certain regions worldwide, or who make certain lifestyle choices, face a higher amount of potentially dangerous environmental factors than those living in areas without such risks. People facing the greatest danger live in communities with excessive solar radiation, eat toxin-tainted foods, drink unsafe water, or get exposed to dangerous pesticides, herbicides, heavy-metal toxins, allergens or other potential carcinogens.

To this point, medical professionals have yet to launch a comprehensive study on how much—if at all—the use of prescribed HGH might lessen or stop the negative impacts of such environmental factors.

Even before such integral studies, we believe that the use of injectable HGH likely would have decreased the risk of diseases and rapid-aging among mature people within those areas. We know from statistical data that children, who almost always possess naturally high HGH levels, suffer a far lower rate of debilitating or fatal diseases than mature people living in the same regions.

Should you fear "free radicals?"

These days the term "free radicals" takes on a much different connotation than it might have during the rebellious, anti-establishment 1960s. Within the medical profession, the "Free Radical Theory" has gained some degree of acceptance along with the "Wear-and-Tear" and "Random Events" theories, contributing at least some to the aging process.

Many of us might remember our high school chemistry class where we learned that a radical—also called a free radical—is an atom, molecule or ion, each with an unpaired electron that results in an open-shell configuration. The result is an imbalanced electrical energy that forces free radicals to attach to other molecules.

Negative environmental factors such as carcinogens or excessive radiation can cause the cells to generate free radicals, creating havoc in the structure of vital proteins, body chemistry and metabolism— thereby creating extensive bodily damage. Worsening matters, free radicals attack cell membranes and create metabolic waste products, including lipofuscins.

Although the word "lipofuscin" might sound like an evil character from the top-selling Harry Potter book series, in real-life biology these substances are wicked metabolic waste products that darken the skin of mature Caucasians—commonly known as those dreaded age spots or liver spots. Even worse, these pigments interfere with our cells' abilities to repair and reproduce themselves, while disturbing RNA and DNA syntheses and destroying vital cellular enzymes necessary for our bodies' vital chemical processes.

We know that far more mature people suffer damage from free radicals than young adults and children. Could the body's natural decrease in HGH among older people increase the likelihood that free radicals will occur in such individuals? We think the answer is "Yes."

Remember, the vast majority of our patients who use injectable HGH are in their 60s, 70s and 80s. These people cry out with joy or at least smile when they discover their liver spots or age spots have disappeared. Such reversals are among primary factors that lead us to believe that this hormone can cease or at least curtail the horrific biological damages that free radicals inflict.

Human bodies lack money-back guarantees

The "Wear-and-Tear Theory" on aging equates your body to a car or machine that eventually breaks down. Alex Comfort, best known for his blockbuster book "The Joy of Sex," described his groundbreaking "Wear-and-Tear Theory" in the 1956 book "The Biology of Senescence," which went into its third printing in the late 1970s.

Comfort proclaimed that through the process of living, the physiology, biochemistry and cellular morphology of the body undergoes natural wear and tear. Under this theory, the nervous, endocrine and vascular systems and connective tissue all suffer specific damage over a period of time.

Think of the classic 1936 film "Modern Times," in which comic actor Charlie Chaplin's beloved character, The Tramp, portrays an assembly line factory worker. The Tramp gets force-fed into a giant feeding machine, his famed little body ravaged by the contraption's many nuts and bolts.

Under Comfort's theory, in a sense your body is like poor Chaplin's when ravaged by the machine, except that your own internal mechanisms cause the damage. Meantime, yet another group of gerontologists blame aging on environmental toxins, cosmic rays, food additives and pesticides, plus contaminates in food and pesticides.

Summary

At present, there is no known "cure" for aging, or an irrefutable Fountain of Youth, yet injectable bio-identical HGH goes a long way toward reversing those characteristics. The mystery of the aging process is a complex puzzle. However, the role of the neuroendocrine system and the recorded decline in the "master hormone" HGH is proving to be a key factor in solving this enigma.

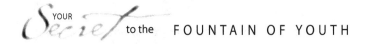

CHAPTER 9

Life's Eternal Tragedy: You were born to die

If the many theories on aging weren't already enough to send you into a deep depression, in a sense at this very moment you're plummeting to your death. At birth, the moment you exited your mother's womb, you were immediately jettisoned from the safety of her body into a free-fall toward your eventual demise.

In this regard, at birth you were like a person thrown from an airplane at 30,000 feet, except here the altitude is 76 years—the average life expectancy, rather than being measured in terms of distance—and you're free falling without a parachute.

Yes, you're still spiraling down and you're going to get old—if your free-fall lasts long enough—and you're going to die, and current technology lacks any cushion or emergency craft whatsoever to permanently stop the fall. Within two years of being thrown into mid-air, you began to speak.

As the ground approached at what seemed an ever-increasing rate, you reached adolescence, your young adult years and eventually middle age. During those phases you paid little or no attention to the eventual and inevitable impact.

Then, suddenly—now—you're approaching the various stages of advanced age or dying, experiencing attributes identified by the late psychiatrist Elisabeth Kübler-Ross, M.D., denial, anger, depression, bargaining and acceptance.

In the bargaining phase, you initially yearn to return to the mother aircraft where you started. Since this is impossible and because the laws of nature prohibit a reversal of time, you want to improve the quality of your remaining free-fall experience and possibly delay the impact or decrease its painfulness at least somewhat.

During the final stages of this amazing experience, you're lucky enough to find a friend, acquaintance or medical professional who explains to you the amazing benefits of injectable HGH. Eager for knowledge, you track down an expert who explains in an easy-to-understand manner how the hormone naturally works when generated by your body and as an injectable substance.

Then, after obtaining a legal prescription, you can begin enjoying the benefits, blessed with a sense that HGH—as an emergency, final-days parachute—could very well lessen the characteristics of aging and pain from the eventual impact.

How your body yearns to make HGH

A serene, tranquil sensation comes to many people as they learn the intricacies of how human growth hormone gets generated by the body. You'd need to memorize a pile of complex, very detailed medical books to learn all the many specifics.

The anterior compartment of the pituitary gland, the size of a large kidney bean at the base of the brain in a bony cavity called the sella turcica, produces the HGH hormone that keep people healthy and vital—giving the ability to grow, heal fast and maintain a youthful appearance.

Adding to its importance, HGH also mobilizes fat stored for fuel, and enhances protein synthesis. Thanks to this function, mature patients who receive injectable HGH in replacement therapy lose body fat and gain muscle, even when treated for a short period of time.

In another area of the brain the hypothalamus, lying above the pituitary, sends out a variety of signals including one called "growth hormone releasing hormone," sometimes called GHRH.

At times, the hypothalamus generates somatostatin, a hormone that temporarily inhibits the production of HGH, a polypeptide hormone

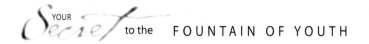

comprised of a long section of 191 amino acids. On command, in order to regulate the body's growth, healing and youthful characteristics, the hypothalamus shuts down somatostatin production, while also sending signals to the pituitary—commanding that it send bursts of active HGH into the body.

HGH surges into the blood stream for brief, intermittent periods, mostly during our deepest sleep, a limited time of rapid-eye movement, characterized by our most vivid dreams. Meantime, the anterior pituitary also secretes a variety of other hormones, including prolactin, a thyroid stimulating hormone, a luteinizing hormone, a follicle stimulating hormone, and an adrenal corticotropic hormone.

Once released into the bloodstream, HGH lasts only a very short period of time, usually a half hour at most. During this period, the liver plays a vital role in transforming the initial HGH that it receives via the blood into another hormone-related substance, commonly known as insulin-like growth factor one or IGF-1.

As the primary and active metabolite of human growth hormone, IGF-1 works on primary endocrine organs such as the thyroid gland, the adrenal glands, and the gonads in both males and females.

When HGH works its "magic"

From the liver, IGF-1 travels to the body's various tissues, giving organs, muscles and bones the ability to grow from infancy through the young adult years. As already noted, these same growth-oriented factors enable the body to heal from wounds, while also keeping the muscles and skin firm and healthy looking.

To keep the body from growing too much, the pituitary gland senses when maximum amounts of HGH are in the bloodstream, and at that point this vital gland shuts down production of the hormone. This also signals to the hypothalamus to stop making GHRH.

Physicians consider HGH as natural rather than synthetic, because the body produces the same hormone. The recombinant form of this hormone, produced in pharmaceutical laboratories, also gets a natural designation because pharmaceutical production companies make it from genetic engineering. At times, some physicians refer to such produced human growth hormone as rGH, the first letter designating "recombinant."

Some medical professionals also use the terms GH or hGH, with the first letter lower-cased. We're among those who downplay the use of such terms, largely because pharmaceutical distributors no longer extract the hormone from pituitaries of cadavers. All along, physicians consider recombinant HGH produced in laboratories as pure or 100-percent free of contaminants.

Discover more interesting details about HGH

To fully understand the power of HGH, it's essential to know how the body's endocrine or glandular system communicates between cells and organs. In order to grasp the process, it's important to understand that the endocrine system serves as an immensely complicated process that encompasses complex biochemical, physiologic and cellular biological applications. First, keep in mind that the endocrine system takes orders from both the central nervous system and the immune system.

These dual functions make understanding the endocrine system's full and comprehensive functions a formidable challenge. From our view, people interested in using injectable HGH should remember that the word "endocrine" means "the internal secretion of biological active substances into the blood stream, in order to regulate the function of

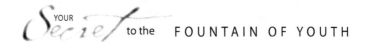

a target organ." Medical professionals and laymen alike refer to these biological substances as hormones.

At this point, it's also vital to understand that as a hormone, HGH is not a steroid. Unlike human growth hormone, steroids are heralded, and rightly so, as potentially harmful substances—especially when injected without proper supervision from a medical professional. HGH hails as among the most notable of eight separate hormones produced by the pituitary.

Various chemical compounds within the body play an essential role in forming the building blocks and creation of hormones. These vital building blocks include proteins and polypeptides, fatty acids, natural steroids produced within the body, and vitamins.

All along, the complex interactions between the endocrine, nervous and immune systems cause vital body functions in a science known to physicians as "neuro-immuno-endocrinology."

Learn about nature's ingenious triggers

Three different mechanisms or triggers play a significant role in the pituitary's release of hormones:

1. **Daily brain interactions:** These functions, sometimes called "circadian rhythms," hinge on essential daily sleep-wake cycles.
2. **Negative feedback interaction:** After a target organ gets an amount of hormone that satisfies its needs, the pituitary stops production of those hormones—temporarily.
3. **Other intervening influences:** Factors such as stress, emotional trauma, nutritional illnesses, infections and other activities in hormonal glands influence the secretion of HGH.

Amid these various processes, the posterior portion of the pituitary receives direct neural stimulation from the hypothalamus—while secreting only two hormones, oxytocin and vasopressin.

Doctors call the normal physiologic decrease in HGH as we age "somatopause," the equivalent of menopause in women and andropause in men. While scientists have yet to proclaim a specific reason for this decline, from our view various factors might contribute, such as a drop in available amino acid precursors necessary for the actual production of HGH within the pituitary gland.

In addition, the hypothalamus might sustain a decrease in its release of stimulatory hormones that generate HGH, while the hormone that inhibits its production—somatostatin—might increase.

The natural decrease in HGH remains inevitable

The body's ability to absorb, digest and assimilate proteins diminishes as people age, losing the ability to absorb protein and proper amounts of hydrochloric acids through digestive enzymes. Called hypochlorhydria, this condition becomes evident in many digestive diseases including diabetes mellitus, hypothyroidism, chronis hepatitis, osteoporosis, and chronic autoimmune malfunctions.

The frequent or chronic use of antacid drug therapy or anti-inflammatory drugs might influence these digestive problems. Also, mature patients sometimes exacerbate these difficulties by reducing their body's production of hydrochloric acid by eating or drinking foods or drinks high in carbohydrates, sugars, alcohol, caffeine and refined meals.

The aging process occasionally results in increased stress or trauma, potentially causing the hypothalamus to lose its ability to manufacture and release growth hormone releasing hormone or GHRH. Adding to the problem, a lack of certain nutrients in the diet might contribute to the downturn in HGH production. In diabetics, high blood sugar levels reduce growth hormone-releasing activity.

In addition, scientists have discovered that in a natural reaction to stress, the body generates glucocorticoid hormones that inhibit the effect of HGH production. And high levels of blood sugars and glucocorticoids stimulate the inhibitory hormone, somatostatin.

Patients enjoy learning these details

With patients, we help make the learning process fun and easy by describing details in an easy-to-understand manner that almost all middle-aged people and seniors can visualize. Let's use our friend David Cartwright as an example.

Just like you did, David's body began producing HGH while still in his mother's womb. For him, this process began at the onset of the embryonic stage within three weeks after his parents conceived him in July 1933.

In the womb and following birth, the growth process happens to all healthy individuals. Like David's body did within his mother, your pituitary gland near the base of the brain began broadcasting to the rest of your tiny body when you were in your mother. Ever since, your brain has pumped out HGH that your entire body craves and needs.

When in his mother's womb, tiny David's entire immature body needed and craved these proverbial HGH signals from his pituitary gland in order to grow enough to live after birth. Without appropriate amounts of these hormones within the womb in the form of HGH, he would have died, resulting in a miscarriage.

To handle this chore, nature provides the hypothalamus just above the pituitary gland. Think of the hypothalamus as your body's expert in giving each organ and cell all the appropriate hormones that each craves and needs.

From the day he was born in April 1934, little David's hypothalamus preferred to blare out 75 percent of his body's essential growth signals during the wee hours of the morning.

The internal vibration station

Tiny David's hypothalamus pumped out vital HGH chemicals, mostly during REM sleep, a normal stage of sleep characterized by rapid eye movements. Most of us reach our deepest sleep during late-night hours or the wee hours of the morning, or within a few hours after we begin our longest period of daily sleep.

Scientists have yet to determine why our internal broadcasting system prefers to pump out its most intense HGH signals during periods of heavy sleep, and the remaining 25 percent through the rest of the day. The strength increases steadily, month-to-month and year-to-year till peaking in our mid-20s.

After initially being produced by the pituitary and released into the blood system, HGH enters the liver—which transforms this substance into the amazing insulin growth factor-1, also known as IGF-1, as previously described. You might want to think of IGF-1 as the speakers that amplify, strengthen or target the vital signals or songs that each cell of the body craves.

Just like all newborns, at birth soft spots riddled the top of David's skull, spaces where the bones had not yet grown together, so that his mother could squeeze him through the birth canal.

Babies better grow

Just three months after David's birth, his father, Carl, boasted to the same neighbor that, "Our new little guy is growing like a weed. Only God could understand how this happens, but I'm proud."

Herein came proof of the miracle of HGH. Without proper amounts of the hormone little David would have died a painful death during his

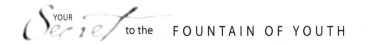

first year free from the womb, and the same horrible fate would have happened to you had your signals during infancy gone haywire.

Proper HGH signals, as mandated by the hypothalamus, cause regulation and growth of nearly every cell and tissue, from childhood through adolescence. Overly rapid growth of any single organ or insufficient growth of some areas of the body could cause fatal organ dysfunction.

By the end of infancy at his first birthday, little David's skull bones had begun to fuse together, lessening the danger of a fatal injury or accidental fall that might cause horrific trauma to the head. As with the vast majority of children, HGH had done its job well.

Understand this amazing system

Thanks to the mysteries of Mother Nature, the HGH-regulating area of the brain—the hypothalamus—knows exactly what hormonal signals to send, at what intensity, and when. During the toddler stage from ages one through three, David learned to walk, talk and go to the bathroom on demand.

Thanks to the natural miracle of HGH, coupled with guidance or examples set by his parents, like most toddlers at 36 months he spoke in cohesive sentences, played different games, knew the difference between genders, anticipated routines, played with toys in imaginative ways, and attempted to sing songs. The growth process enabled David's brain to develop on schedule.

As we know, sadly or at least as biology intended, David already was pre-programmed to slow down during middle age, show signs of aging and eventually die—preferably well after age 50. But before that all could happen, he first needed to grow at the predictable schedule, largely because humans are programmed to achieve physical and sexual maturity in order to repopulate the Earth.

David evolved through early childhood as predicted from ages four through six. An only child, he entered the first grade in the fall of 1940.

Seemingly as if in a science fiction movie, each night during David's deepest sleep the mysterious and life-giving HGH signals continued to course through his body, more than at any other time of day. By preadolescence from ages 9-12, for the first time David developed an attitude of self-identity and independence, plus a sense of responsibility such as handling chores and envisioning a future career. Human growth hormone helped make all this possible.

Those gangly pre-teen and teen years

Just as yours did, David's hypothalamus and pituitary gland conducted a symphony of work behind the scenes from the beginning of his elementary school days through high school. Like cymbals conducted to clang at an exact, precise second during a symphony, his final baby teeth popped out during reading time in first grade class.

The many wonders of HGH worked magic for him, pushing in his adult teeth straight and true, and hard enough—hopefully—to last a lifetime. At age 9, David suffered a fractured right leg when he stupidly drove his bicycle in front of a cruising Buick Roadmaster. Right away, the hypothalamus and pituitary put David's internal HGH production and distribution into a crescendo mode, and just less than six weeks later the fracture had fully healed.

Those mystical internal signals skipped at a natural and predictable off-beat mode at ages 13-15, when some of David's limbs and physical characteristics seemed either too big or too small for the rest of his burgeoning body. A keen observer might conclude that the confounding hypothalamus was off kilter, as vital gland's natural skills had gone awry. Yet all went well, just as the case with other young teens thanks to the great powers of HGH.

David's voice cracked on occasion during this period as his body transformed from that of a boy into the frame of a strong, strapping young man. He never told his parents this, but starting at age 14, about a year after pubic hair spouted around his testicles, his body began confusing him, displaying the sexual characteristics of adulthood. Without even consulting with Fred's external thought process, HGH had started to play a supposed trick on him, right on schedule.

The hypothalamus' wicked humor

Just as they do for many young guys, David's internal hormones forced him to reach his most active sexual capacity well before he ever enjoyed intimate relations for the first time. At David's 18th birthday in his family's back yard in April 1952, all he could think about were the women his own age and the sensual things he would like to do with them. Typically mischievous, the hypothalamus played this signal about every 30 seconds, driving David wild with desire—as Mother Nature demands.

This continued the following June, on the day David scurried to the local Marine Corps recruiting office without first consulting his parents, Carl and Betty. He joined on the spot, incurring the wrath of his folks. An only child, by mid-summer David got shipped off to boot camp. In mid-November, he began serving on the front lines in the Korean War.

Thanks to HGH, David's body was already pulsating with boundless energy, and strapping muscles by the time he reached basic training. His V-shaped frame and strength adapted well to vigorous, regimentary routines. This put him in perfect physical condition in time for the Battle for Pork Chop Hill in 1953, when a sniper's bullet cruelly ripped through a fleshy area just below his right shoulder. On the spot, medics worked feverishly to stop his profuse bleeding.

Since David's hypothalamus didn't want to die either, this amazing gland feverishly worked overtime. The vital talents of this organ paid off, rejuvenating vital muscles, blood vessels and even some significant nerve endings.

The hypothalamus is an expert at growth, enabling cells to differentiate, rejuvenate and repair. David's wound undoubtedly would have killed a much older man who lacks the maximum amounts of naturally produced HGH.

Those hits just keep on coming

Like it does for many young men on the cusp of their third decade, the hypothalamus also continued pumping anabolic hormones into David at age 19 when he returned home to his worried family. At exactly 6 feet, he was a full two inches taller than on high school graduation day. And by age 20, HGH added on another inch for good measure.

Following an early honorable military discharge due to his war wound, at his parents urging, David entered New York University in the fall semester. There, he joined the wrestling team and promptly suffered a broken nose, which the hypothalamus soon repaired to its original prominent stature. HGH continues to exert its effect on the repair of bone and supporting tissues throughout life, particularly during the first 2 ½ decades.

Amid his engineering studies, a plethora of HGH gave young David the energy and seemingly endless zest to hit the books, work a part-time job, and party around the clock. Thanks to HGH, sleep didn't seem to matter. Do you remember when your internal HGH-band broadcast station gave you similar pep and vigor, seemingly enough spunk to tackle just about any challenge?

Somehow the hormone enabled him to find the time to amass bonds or friendships with numerous young women. Finally, David lost his virginity. That night, the hypothalamus went into overdrive, as if he and this gland had worked their entire lives to prepare David's body for this moment—and indeed, that was the very case.

Since the sexual urge reigns as one of the most powerful internal and natural drives, the hypothalamus had paid lots of attention to this aspect of David's physical make-up. Each time, always excited and eager, David responded the way nature told him to, culminating in a blast off that would have made the then-burgeoning NASA program proud.

HGH helps spark romance

David and Pamela Galloway fell in love within a week after they met for the first time at NYU on campus in April 1957, the day after his 23rd birthday. At age 19, thanks to her own hypothalamus' focus on the female gender, Pamela's hips were firm and round, accenting her taught, muscular waist. Her internal hormone mechanisms created full, firm breasts, and the sight of him ignited her passion.

Par for customs dictated by the times, the couple started dating that summer when their hormone glands did everything possible to motivate them to mate. Morals and personal preferences enabled them to overcome natural urges as they gyrated that summer away, often dancing to popular current tunes from Elvis and Buddy Holly to the Big Bopper.

David's hypothalamus made him fantasize about Pamela night and day. His naturally high and persistent HGH gave no relief, pumping appropriate amounts of hormones.

Pamela broke into tears and said "yes" right away, as soon as David proposed to her in October 1957 in Central Park after they enjoyed chocolate shakes at a nearby malt shop. Pamela's hormones sent sparks of anticipation roaring through her body. Unlike her fiancée, at the time she was a virgin, and HGH made her libido soar.

Enjoy the peak period

Four weeks after David earned a bachelor's degree in civil engineering, he and Pamela were married at Saint Patrick's Cathedral in New York City in June 1958. Like many young people, their bodies responded the way nature commands that night while making love till sunrise.

Do you remember your young adult years, when able to share such non-stop joy and passion? Just like you have, in the years and decades that followed Pamela and David showed a significant decrease in both their desire and ability for such intense lovemaking, largely because their internal HGH production tapered off to a small percentage of its former maximum levels.

Shortly after their wedding, though, in denial of their pending old age and eventual deaths, HGH enabled Pamela and David to tackle many of life's most formidable challenges. You see, eight days after the newlyweds returned from their honeymoon, David's father died of a sudden cardiac arrest while working at his accounting firm, exactly 25 years to the day after David was conceived.

Back in 1933 when David was conceived, his father reigned as a vibrant stud thanks to his own hypothalamus and pituitary gland. Yet par for the course as dictated by Mother Nature, Carl's HGH levels dropped off dramatically in his 30s, 40s and early 50s, contributing to his deteriorating heart function and leading to his eventual demise.

The mystery of early maturity

By our estimates, David's internal HGH levels reached their maximum amounts on or about August 1959, when the measurable amounts of the hormone pulsated through his bloodstream at a predictable and measurably high level of 347. Average men attain maximum IGF-1 levels of 300-350 while in their mid-20s, while the level of IGF-1 for women peaks at 250-300.

and nerves in what medical professionals call a "negative feedback interaction."

Just as yours did in your 30s, this relationship among the body's internal systems begins to function with much less efficiency than just a decade earlier. Once these automatic "on" and "off" switches start going haywire, many vital organs throughout the body begin receiving less vital HGH than necessary, sometimes getting the hormone at the wrong times or failing to receive adequate supplies when needed most.

For both David and his late father, these steadily decreasing inefficiencies lowered good cholesterol, worsened cardiac function, put blood pressure off kilter, and weakened their abilities to ward off coronary artery disease.

Exacerbating the problem, the efficiency of HGH depends largely on the complex endocrine or glandular system of the body—which, during good health, communicates complex and important information among cells and organs.

At age 39 David suffered a mild heart attack while at his job as a civil engineer. An ambulance crew rushed him to a hospital, where physicians blamed coronary artery disease rather than pinpointing the underlying reason, the decreased efficiency of his HGH distribution.

When in good health, complex interactions occur between the glandular, nervous and immune systems. Various compounds within the body generate hormones from essential proteins, polypeptides, fatty acids, amino acids, steroids and vitamins. All these integral systems had started going off kilter within David's body—which just 20 years earlier had been at the peak of efficiency, saving him from potential death from his war wound.

By the time David reached 61 and Pamela was 57, the couple had not made love for a full three years, due largely to their natural decrease in

HGH, each having lost enough significant interest to "give it a try." Our tests would have shown that by this point David's HGH distribution had lost more than 50 percent of its former peak efficiency. Pamela's growth hormone levels had slid way downhill as well.

On Labor Day that year, this couple's 35-year-old sons, Carl and Kevin, each visited David and Pamela's home. By this point the twins sported similar-size pot bellies, each more than a decade past his HGH prime. The family enjoyed a lavish summer barbecue, while David and Pamela's seven grandchildren—ages 5 through 12—scurried about the back yard, all of their young bloodstreams overflowing with HGH.

Summary

While we're all destined to die, the aging process is predictable and inevitable if we live long enough to experience the characteristics of old age.

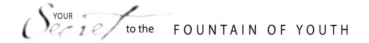

CHAPTER 10

News Flash: Acquire and administer your HGH prescription

For many people, the aging and dying process brings to mind the longtime observation that "Watching an old man die is like seeing a library burn." Yet an increase in the popularity of HGH could soon change such public perceptions, at least in terms of enabling seniors to enjoy a better quality of life until they die.

Despite the inevitable aging process, significant medical advances involving HGH have enabled mature people like Pamela and David to thrive and prosper physically and emotionally during their golden years. The many benefits this couple enjoys today would not have been possible for their own parents.

By the mid-1970s, physicians began injecting HGH that had been extracted from cadavers into children who were dwarfs; the youngsters' bodies had produced insufficient amounts of the hormone for them to grow to average heights. Many of these children initially benefited.

However, by the early 1980s, some of these children began suffering from a viral dementia, a complication caused by contaminated HGH. Partly in order to reverse the problem, scientists developed or expanded technology enabling them to produce the hormone in sterile laboratories on a massive scale rather than extracting the substance from cadavers. Recombinant DNA technology kicked into gear during the mid-1980s.

During production, scientists isolate and amplify DNA or genes, before injecting them with precision into another cell, creating a transgenic—or genetically engineered—bacterium. This hormone creates seemingly perfect replications of this vital substance, the exact replica, 191-chain polypeptide, is produced.

Why are injections necessary?

Naturally, many patients receiving HGH prescriptions for the first time wonder why they must administer the hormone via injection, rather than orally with pills or even by drinking liquids. We tell all patients that—other when possibly using certain oral sprays—the digestive process breaks down the vital, working characteristics of HGH that would have made it effective in the body.

Remember that when produced naturally, HGH is a 191-amino acid, single-chain polypeptide or protein hormone. Hydrogen, oxygen, nitrogen and carbon create a chain of amino acids, longer than the majority of molecular characteristics displayed by other hormones. Your digestive system—except possibly when using certain oral sprays—cannot absorb these long chains from the HGH in their original forms because of acid and enzyme degradation.

Hydrochloric acid within the stomach would cleave or break up the essential amino acids. The digestive process would prevent any viable HGH from getting to the liver, a vital step in the body's process of creating IGF-1, the working component of HGH.

Perhaps someday medical experts will be able to develop HGH-laden slow-release capsules or pellets that physicians can insert or implant into your body. Then, your metabolism would slowly absorb the capsules in a time-release system, similar in many ways to a process that physicians now use to treat prostate cancer or long-acting birth control hormones.

For patients receiving HGH, this would eliminate the need to administer injections from three to six times weekly, while also ending the hassle of transporting injectable forms of the substance in cool or refrigerated containers when traveling.

Learn vital basics

Upon getting your first legal prescription for injectable human growth hormone, you'll need to know basics on everything from costs to acquisition methods, plus mixing necessary substances, administering injections, and storing HGH while traveling.

Average costs: Most patients with prescriptions for injectable HGH spend $400-$600 per month for this natural substance. That comes out to $4,800 to $7,200 per year. Each person's exact cost depends on how much the physician prescribes or recommends, or on the amounts the patient can afford or wants to use within parameters of what is prescribed.

A majority of adult patients must pay for HGH themselves. Medicare, Medicaid and insurance companies only authorize these payments for adults needing treatment for any one of three specific types of FDA-approved uses: AIDS wasting, adult-short bowel syndrome, and the continuation of childhood HGH deficiency syndrome.

The cost usually averages out to about $25 per injection, and most patients receive from three to six injections per week. Some patients write off these purchase expenses on their U.S. income taxes at amounts the government allows for each income bracket for health care-related costs.

Delivery methods: After receiving a prescription for injectable human growth hormone, the substance usually is dispensed by a compounding pharmacy—rather than from a standard pharmacy such as at Wal-Mart®. Pharmacists or physicians at compounding pharmacies use long-standing processes to mix drugs or substances to fit a patient's unique needs.

Most patients have their injectable HGH delivered at home via FedEx® or UPS®, usually in amounts just enough to last for one month. The potency of unused HGH decreases after 30 days.

Mix ingredients: When you receive HGH it's usually sent in an un-reconstituted form, one vial containing powder and a separate vial of liquid. After receiving proper training or instructions from a physician or from a compounding pharmacy, you must mix contents from the vials. The resulting mixture usually is placed into other vials, each holding up to 10 milliliters.

Inject yourself

Anyone initially concerned about the process of injecting themselves with HGH has little to worry about. Our many patients tell us there is minimal pain, and among those of us in the Forsythe family using HGH we've never felt any discomfort. Here are basics you need to know about self-injection:

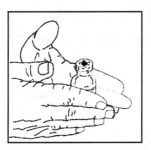 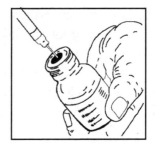

- **Quick process:** While careful to conduct each step the right way, the entire task usually takes less than a few minutes. Most physicians give their first-time clients fast and easy lessons on this process at the time these patients receive initial prescriptions.

- **Injection time:** Always administer injections late at night, or shortly before bedtime. The body absorbs HGH best during your deepest sleep, commonly called the rapid-eye-movement or REM period.

- **Environment:** Choose a private well-lighted place so that you can see clearly. Administer injections when alone, out of sight from children in order to avoid sparking their curiosity.
- **Handle syringe:** First, push out any air that might be in the syringe. Then, pull back the syringe pump, sucking air into the device. Stop at the indicator showing the dosage you need, such as one milliliter or two milliliters.
- **Displace air:** Push the needle through the small "bulls-eye" in the center of a rubber diaphragm on the vial, and then inject the air into the vial containing HGH.
- **Fill syringe:** Invert the positions of the syringe and the vial, so that the container is now on top. Then, pull back the syringe pump to the amount of your prescribed dosage.
- **Administer injection:** Poke the needle fully into your belly fat or love handle at or around the sides of your waistline. There is rarely any pain when this is done right. People with little or no belly fat can inject at their rumps or fatty areas of their thighs.
- **Restore material:** Right after completing the injection, replace any remaining HGH back into the refrigerator while still in the vial.

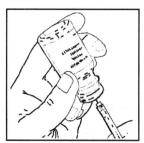 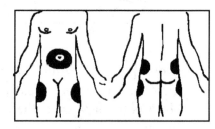

Recommended storage methods

Because the effectiveness of injectable human growth hormone decreases at room temperature, you should store your HGH and syringes in a refrigerator. If possible, use a compartment that children have difficulty finding or reaching.

When traveling, take your HGH in a refrigerated or cool container, packed inside check-in luggage. Avoid taking your prescriptions inside carry-on luggage or purses in order to avoid unnecessary questioning from authorities.

Carry your prescription note

To prevent any unwarranted accusations, keep your prescription papers or a physician's permission slip on hand, in case you're stopped by airport security personnel or even by a traffic cop. If you're stopped and searched, be sure to tell authorities that HGH and syringes are legal when prescribed by a physician and obtained from the state where that medical professional practices medicine. Remember, injectable HGH is illegal when obtained via the Internet or when sent direct to you from other countries.

Number of weekly doses

Injections are usually given once daily, and the most a physician prescribes is six injections per week. This gives the pituitary gland the opportunity during a full day each week to continue its own natural production of HGH without benefit of injections—and enabling the gland to remain active on its own.

Lots of patients start their treatment regimens at five or six injections per week, before tapering off to three or four weekly. This course of action often is used for either or both of two reasons:

1. **Conditioning:** At the start, get your body used to these injections, before cutting back to lower levels.
2. **Economy:** Some patients request the lower frequencies for financial reasons.

Although these basics are easy to learn and implement, be sure to do them all the right way. From the start, make a habit of using these

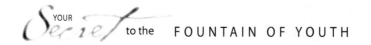

YOUR FOUNTAIN OF YOUTH

suggested procedures. This way you can position yourself to get the greatest benefit from your prescription.

Production will accelerate

More than a dozen manufacturing facilities worldwide produce enough injectable HGH for an estimated 160,000 Americans, with each patient spending an average $6,000 yearly for the hormone. That brings the current annual industry to around $1 billion, a total that we foresee booming to $100 billion or perhaps even $1 trillion within a decade.

By some estimates, at least 7,900 Baby Boomers in the United States reach age 60 every day, or a whopping 2.8 million people per year. If just 5 percent—approximately 140,000 individuals per year—start receiving injectable HGH, the total expenditures could easily grow by a minimum $1 billion yearly.

Of course, these totals pale by comparison to the overall world population, estimated in mid-2008 at 6.68 billion. At the current average prices of about $25 per injection, a vast majority of people from other nations would lack resources to obtain injectable HGH.
As with other pharmaceutical products, we anticipate that the overall worldwide price per dose will decrease significantly from current levels as burgeoning overall demand generates increased production. These price changes should gradually click into gear as distribution intensifies.

Meantime, we expect demand within the USA to double, triple or even surge to far greater levels by mid-2010, especially after word spreads of the conspiracy to keep you from knowing the truth about injectable HGH.

A Major Issue: Off-label prescriptions

While it's obvious to some people, many consumers would benefit by

148

knowing the definition and importance of off-label prescriptions. This seems especially vital, since most HGH prescriptions are for off-label treatment of anti-aging characteristics. When a physician or medical professional gives a prescription "off-label," the substance, device or drug gets issued as a treatment different from those authorized by the federal government.

Medical professionals insist the practice of giving off-label prescriptions seems widespread. By some estimates, about 60 percent of U.S. domestic legal drug distribution in any given year is issued off-label. This especially holds true with HGH, since the only authorized direct use of the hormone is for dwarfism, AIDS wasting and lower tract digestive problems. When prescribing HGH as treatment for anti-aging, physicians or medical professionals are issuing "off-label" orders to pharmacies.

"The Physicians Desk Reference™," a book considered the proverbial bible on pharmaceuticals for medical professionals, clearly indicates that physicians can issue off-label prescriptions for virtually any of the many thousands of drugs it describes. There is no ethical problem issuing off-label prescriptions, and merely issuing drugs "off-label" does not constitute malpractice. In an oncology practice, between 70 percent and 80 percent of prescriptions are written "off-label."

From our view, the issuance of HGH as an off-label treatment to a mature patient with low natural levels of the hormone is proper, ethical and highly advised. Part of the issue in the government's attempted prosecution of me hinged at least in part on the fact that I had issued the hormone off-label to an undercover federal agent—although the man's blood test clearly indicated he had insufficient amounts of natural HGH in his body.

An illegal or underground market

According to some official estimates, at least 30,000 licensed medical professionals nationwide prescribe injectable HGH. We believe the actual number of distributors approaches 50,000 or perhaps much more. Many doctors distribute the hormone covertly or surreptitiously in order to stay out of range from the public radar. Since my trial, case law has established that it is a legal precedence.

In the past, a growing number of Internet sites have offered HGH in a wide variety of forms and distribution methods including an oral-spray that we consider far less effective than injectable HGH. So, keep in mind that federal or state laws make obtaining HGH illegal unless prescribed by an appropriate licensed medical professional and obtained within the state where the prescription was issued.

A percentage of medical professionals who legally issue such prescriptions are homeopaths that practice forms of alternative medicine, licensed in only a limited number of states including Nevada, Arizona and Connecticut. Professionals licensed to practice naturopathy—which emphasizes the ability of the body to heal and maintain itself—can prescribe HGH in states including Washington, Oregon and California.

As you might imagine, the laws on HGH are murky from state to state. For instance, by some accounts a doctor of Oriental medicine would be breaking the law if he prescribed HGH in one state, but the same professional could issue a perfectly legal prescription for the same substance in another state if he holds a license there for that profession.

Summary

Patients should follow various prescribed methods and procedures when acquiring, administering and storing injectable HGH—under the supervision of a qualified and licensed medical professional.

CHAPTER 11

Some results indicate HGH precursor sprays work

To this point, injectable HGH has continued to remain what we call the "gold standard," the premiere, most acceptable and most effective form for administering the hormone. However, the average monthly cost of about $500-$600 for this method has discouraged some potential users from even trying the hormone.

Yet good news has emerged in the cost issue, at least from the view of at least some medical professionals. The fee is now as little as $49.95 monthly or perhaps even less, for Lipotropin™, an oral spray that some physicians consider effective. Thanks to research and development by numerous medical professionals, especially by a widely acclaimed physician, Mark Gordon, M.D., amino acid complexes are available as a spray.

Based on Doctor Gordon's findings, some patients might consider Lipotropin™ "a good second choice" to the more expensive injectable HGH. At least until more research or developments are completed, we consider the injectable form of HGH as far more preferable.

Whether you seek HGH in what we consider the most recommend form—via injection—or with a spray, always seek the guidance of a licensed physician or homeopath beforehand. Only qualified medical professionals can determine if you need such supplements or treatments, and you'll need these experts to monitor your results.

Patients wishing to take this oral spray should first seek a physical examination and the advice of a medical professional. Although you can purchase Lipotropin™ on a non-prescription basis, the medical professional should be able to recommend a place or method to purchase this product.

Various distributors of Lipotropin™ supply information that indicates this product is a "stimulator" in having the body generate the production of HGH. Some Lipotropin™ distributors tell users to shake the containers, before applying two full sprays under the tongue in the mornings and four sprays just before going to bed.

At least some initial research conducted early in this century indicated that Lipotropin™ increased the body's production of IGF-1—the vital and necessary precursor of HGH—among various individuals who initially had low levels of IGF-1 in a 30-day trial. But among patients who initially had IGF-1 levels that were considered high, in some instances the body decreased or suppressed the amounts of this vital substance.

Binding proteins serve a key function

All along in healthy youngsters and young adults, a related substance, IGFBP-3, plays an integral and related role in generating or distributing IGF-1. In this case the "BP" designates "binding proteins." Also called "carrier proteins," these transport specific substances to various locations within the body. In medical terms, IGFBP-3 is a secretagogue, something that causes another substance to be secreted into the body.

After initial research on Lipotropin™, follow-up studies indicated the need to monitor the levels of IGFBP-3 levels in patients, and the percentage of body fat as well. According to some research, people with excessive percentages of body fat apparently have lower natural release and production of growth hormones.

However, complicating matters, some medical experts consider these initial results as inaccurate because of measuring issues in determining the levels of IGF-1. This, in turn, leads some physicians to avoid concluding that HGH oral sprays are effective in all instances.

Based on study results, some medical professionals concluded that besides growth hormone and IGF-1, various substances including estrogens and Quercetin® help the body to increase IGFBP-3 levels. If correct, some patients might consider this an excellent development, especially because Quercetin® is readily available—seemingly on an over-the-counter basis without prescriptions for as little as 50 capsules at less than $12.

Once again, we feel the urgent need to stress the importance of consulting a licensed medical professional before taking any estrogens or substances in the hopes of increasing the body's level of HGH. Any misuse of pharmaceutical products could lead to adverse side affects or even physical impairments.

Also, at all times, please remember that injectable HGH remains what we consider the "gold standard" method of increasing the levels of these hormones in mature people.

Research indicates positive results

Adding to the complexity of this issue, some medical experts also have concluded that DHEA or dehydroepiandrosterone can play an integral role in increasing the body's levels of IGFBP-3 and IGF-1. As a multi-functional steroid, DHEA impacts a wide range of biological functions—including the hypothalamus, the organ within the brain which is integral to the natural production of HGH.

Hailed as a nanoliposomal secretagogue featuring an amino acid complex, such treatments should be administered or prescribed only by a licensed medical professional. Some results indicate that the greatest increases in IGFBP-3 and IGF-1 levels occur within the first 30 days of starting to use such treatments.

Also, keep in mind that even among the best or most experienced medical experts, measuring the body's levels of estrogens, somatostatin, HGH, IGF-1 and IGFBP-3 can prove difficult.

Remember, the body accelerates or decreases the varying levels of these specific natural substances, depending on an individual person's needs at any given time. Most physicians consider the interaction or inter-working synergy of all these varying substances as highly complex. High amounts of a single hormone or substance might cause the body to lower another amino acid, hormone or estrogen, triggering a natural chain of events.

Such monitoring differences have motivated physicians like Doctor Gordon to stress the importance of administering the amino acid complex nanoliposomal only within the parameters of measurement levels that physicians consider as natural. In medical terms, this means that physicians should strive to maintain levels of each substance within patients at physiological levels—meaning the amounts found in nature.

The impact of HGH spray seems multi-faceted

When administering injectable HGH, medical professionals can determine or measure specific benefits that result from an increase in IGF-1—the precursor to human growth hormone. By contrast, at least based on published reports, the body's ability to produce or increase IGF-1 levels when using oral sprays hinges on the necessity to manipulate a variety of hormones. Largely for this reason, once again we feel a need to stress that from our perspective the injectable form remains the "gold standard" despite the higher costs involved.

As with all medical procedures, physicians or homeopaths should monitor individual patients before, during and after such procedures.

Also, keep in mind that the nanoliposomal secretagogue for HGH oral sprays, which features an amino acid complex, can contain a variety of substances that include:

- **Ornithine**: According to at least one study, when taken orally this amino acid can increase the body's levels of growth hormones.

- **Arginine**: An amino acid found naturally in everything from dairy products to seafood and granola, when taken orally as a possible IGF-1 stimulator this gives a variety of conflicting results—at least based on various studies. Whether individuals receive arginine while active or at rest might play integral roles in ultimate results. From our view, more studies seem necessary on this aspect.

- **Dual roles**: At least one study indicates that prescribed doses of ornithine and arginine when taken together—and with a high-density strength training program—can result in a leaner body mass and strength increases.

- **Other substances:** A variety of other substances including a derivative of a glutaric acid organic compound, which—either individually or when combined—might help increase the body's growth hormone and IGF-1 levels.

- **Digestion**: Some studies indicate that the body can digest and absorb the vital substances from within the nanoliposomal secretagogue. If these findings are correct, this combination might surmount the problem of the body's ability to absorb certain HGH-related oral sprays.

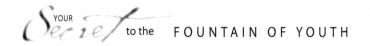

Summary

While from our view injectable HGH remains the much-preferred "gold standard" despite the higher prices of $500-$600 per month, some studies indicate certain HGH sprays for as little as $49.95 per month or possibly less might effectively increase the body's levels of the human growth hormone or of IGF-1, the natural precursor to HGH. Whether seeking injectable HGH or an oral spray, patients should seek advice and regular monitoring from certified and licensed medical professionals.

What they don't want you to know about HGH

CHAPTER 12

How to obtain legal prescriptions of injectable HGH

In all instances, we encourage you to obey the law when seeking and subsequently obtaining injectable HGH. To begin this search, you can contact The American Board of Anti-Aging Medicine or the American Anti-Aging Association; each organization maintains a lengthy list of licensed practitioners. You also can check the yellow pages section of your phone books under the listings of anti-aging physicians.

After selecting one or several licensed professionals to contact, ask them basic background questions. Can the practitioner legally issue prescriptions for injectable HGH within the state where he or she practices medicine? Also inquire about experience, the types of testing this professional requires before issuing a prescription, and whether the professional has ever given prescriptions to people of your gender within your age group.

Once you get an appointment for an initial visit, the cost for that first exam usually ranges from about $150-$300. Unless seeking a prescription for dwarfism, AIDS wasting or specific lower intestine problems, most standard insurance companies plus Medicare or Medicaid refuse to pay for the actual prescription of HGH. A vast majority of people must pay out-of-pocket from their own cash for this phase of the ongoing process.

Add to these costs an additional $200-$450 that you'll need to pay out-of-pocket for medical tests, necessary for the medical professional to determine if your body's HGH levels have decreased enough to justify issuing such a prescription.

For the standard blood tests, licensed professionals look for IGF-1 levels below 300-350 in males and 250-300 in females, the maximum amounts that their bodies produced as young adults. In addition to

157

blood tests, some practitioners also require 24-hour urine tests, measuring the amount of HGH that passes through the body in a full day.

A wide variety of other intricate tests for measuring HGH levels also are possible but not necessarily required. At our clinic, for instance, we give the blood tests at the very minimum and also urine tests.

Is the price worth the results?

Sadly, many seniors on low incomes never will have financial resources to obtain injectable HGH on a regular basis. With average costs ranging about $6,000 per year, the expenses remain far too high for many mature people to even consider. This leaves only a percentage of seniors with the ability to make such treatments an option.

According to the Employee Benefit Research Institute, the total wealth of average Americans reaching or just past normal retirement age grew almost 85 percent in the 10-year period from 1992-2002—at $435,072, up from $235,514. But the same study showed that other seniors had significant declines or losses of all their total wealth.

Numerous studies show a sharp spread in the diversity of wealth in households of older Americans. By some accounts, 10 percent of mature people have 2,500 times as much wealth as the same percentage of seniors with the lowest amount of assets.

Thus, of the 2.8 million Baby Boomers reaching senior status each year, a tenth of them would easily have the means to go on HGH regimes for the remainder of their lives. By our estimates perhaps an additional 10-30 percent of seniors could afford at least some form of an HGH regimen, in some cases if only on a limited basis.

The noted British essayist William Hazlitt proclaimed in the early 1800s that "to be happy, we must be true to nature, and carry our old age along with us." But with the advent of major improvements in medical technology, his proclamations ring an off-key tone, at least for many older people.

Like making car payments

Economists say that average monthly car payments have ballooned above $500 since 2007. So, in monetary terms, for many seniors the decision on obtaining HGH mirrors the choice of whether to buy a new car.

Some mature people might ask themselves questions like: "Do I already have too many vehicles, or would I be willing and able to forego having a car in order to feel more vibrant and healthy for the rest of my life?"

Adding spice to the mix, some seniors might consider trying HGH for a limited period, just to see if it'll give them the boost in vitality and various hoped-for physical improvements. Then, after checking results, they could decide whether to continue treatments.

Still other seniors might choose to sell off limited assets such as an older, seldom-used vehicle in order to amass the $6,000 average yearly expense. This way they could wait until after taking the hormone for a full year before making a final decision. For you, the choice must hinge on your personal desire and financial situation.

To wealthy couples like Fred and Alice, the decision seemed easy thanks to his sizable retirement income. As an overall sector of our population, many mature people are likely to find themselves in a quandary during the next several years as the popularity of HGH booms. Lots of seniors will end up using the common sense or wisdom that they've amassed through their many years.

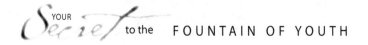

Avoid steep drug prices

Many economists agree that Americans pay more for pharmaceuticals than people in any other country. For instance, in mid-2008 a single 90-pill supply of the cholesterol drug Lipitor® cost $335-$361, according to various surveys. Coupled with the steep prices of other drugs, the average annual prescription drug costs paid by mature people or their insurance companies sometimes exceeds $10,000 or much more.

According to the "Washington Post," the U.S. Customs Bureau estimates that 10 million Americans receive their drugs from other countries in order to lower costs. Meantime, large pharmaceutical companies argue that they must impose high prices in order to pay for vital but expensive research.

Well, imagine the wrath of these huge companies—which we call Big Pharma—once legal and natural HGH gets thrown into the mix. In instances where the hormone would decrease, reverse or remove any adverse characteristics of aging, how much potential revenue would these conglomerate companies lose? For now, we're unaware of any formal economic study on the impact HGH will have on Big Pharma in coming years.

Yet even without such research, these mega-companies already work hard to encourage our government to enable Big Pharma to impose high prices on consumers. The non-partisan Center for Public Integrity reports that Big Pharma spent what we consider a whopping $855 million from 1998-2006 for thousands of Washington, D.C., lobbyists.

So, with all these factors in mind, when considering whether to spend an average $6,000 per year on HGH, you might want to ponder whether such expenditures would help offset or decrease your long-term medical costs.

Summary

Getting a legitimate, legal prescription for injectable HGH within the United States is relatively easy for seniors who can afford the average $500 monthly expense, which comes to about $6,000 per year. Only about 30 percent of today's seniors can readily afford such payments. Some mature people consider lifestyle changes such as cutting back on vacation cruises in order to fit injectable HGH into their annual budgets. We predict that HGH-acquisition costs will decrease somewhat—perhaps 50 percent or even more—as worldwide production surges as a result of increased demand.

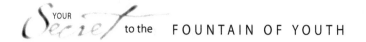

CHAPTER 13

Important: Take Positive Action to Achieve or Maintain Good Health

Like everyone else in the mature population, seniors who use injectable HGH should take care of themselves to help ensure vibrant health well into extreme old age. Diverse and important lifestyle choices ranging from diet to exercise play key roles in achieving or retaining youthful characteristics. Among primary activities, foods or diets we recommend:

- **Vitamins:** Take daily doses of vitamins, essential for maintaining good health throughout the body and organs. We stress the need for all primary vitamins, plus anti-oxidants and minerals including selenium, zinc, phosphorous and magnesium. Calcium, necessary along with vitamin D for absorption in fighting bone deterioration, is essential to both genders, especially women. Men comprise only 10-15 percent of patients suffering from osteoporosis, the severe thinning of bones.

- **Foods:** As an oncology practice, we have extensive experience in recommending anti-cancer meals or foods that promote good overall health. We stress the importance of the three "Bs," beans, Brussels sprouts and broccoli, plus the three "Cs," carrots, cabbage and cauliflower.

Seniors should cut down on milk products and avoid cancer-promoting food, especially red meats, cured ham, salami and pepperoni. Instead, while also avoiding fried selections, mature people should eat more fish and fowl. Healthy diets restrict or curtail foods loaded with simple sugars such as cookies, pies, cake, ice cream or confections of various sorts.

- **Healthy juices:** At our practice, for patients who want, we recommend healthy smoothies that we also recommend they prepare at home on a regular basis. Most of these recipes include soy milk, non-fat yogurt, berries such as blueberries, blackberries or strawberries, bananas and a raw egg, plus a couple tablespoons of flaxseed oil and whey protein. Many patients consider such smoothies delicious, and they're also good for digestion.

- **Exercise:** We refrain from recommending extremely stressful or overly vigorous activities, such as fast-paced marathons that can cause severe wear and tear on muscles and joints. Seniors on treadmills never need quick-paced rates of between 2.5 and 3.5 miles per hour for extensive periods. Instead, we recommend limiting the pace to 3 ½ miles per hour in 30- to 45-minute daily spans up to five days a week. This enables seniors to move muscles and joints. Also, lifting weights, stretching, and enjoying pilates can become extremely important.

"Do not overdo exercise," we tell patients, while also recommending a variety of physical activities such as yoga, biofeedback, meditation and stretching.

- **Sleep:** Seniors who take HGH often report they resume the ability to sleep for lengthy periods of up to eight hours or more at a stretch at night. Many also tell us they start enjoying and recalling multi-color dreams just as they did as children and as young adults. As people age they sleep less at night, sometimes as little as six hours at a stretch. But sleeping longer is better, partly because good, deep sleep is essential in the body's vital healing process. Therefore, we tell seniors taking HGH to enjoy the benefits and sleep for as long as they can.

- **Hobbies:** Thanks partly to their increase in energy, many seniors taking HGH are able to adopt or resume interest in hobbies.

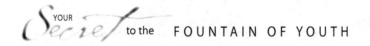
Such activities often enable people to increase their vigor for life, giving them greater reason to live. Potential interests can range from arts and crafts to playing relatively light sports such as golf or low-impact tennis. Many seniors consider gardening and caring for plants extremely rewarding.

- **Faith, religion or spiritual beliefs:** From our perspective, people who lack faith in God or a loving creator have less interest in enjoying vibrant, healthy lives. Attending church or scheduled spiritual services, or even praying alone, often makes seniors feel more vibrant or fulfilled, as if they sense having become more whole or complete.

- **Philanthropy:** Many patients, especially seniors, tell us they feel better about themselves and about the world when they're able to give without reservation to others. Potential options range from giving financially to a worthy cause to volunteering at a hospital for the needy.

Summary

Seniors who take HGH enhance their lives and their health by adopting and implementing sensible exercise and food selections. We strongly advise all our mature patients to take these measures, adding value to their investment in the hormone.

CHAPTER 14

Our clinical results pulverize negative comments

On the strength of consistent and positive clinical test results, we're able to shoot down negative comments from prognosticators who insist the benefits are minimal at best for seniors taking injectable HGH. Some of these negative people—most with little or no experience at prescribing the hormone—claim injectable HGH causes negative side effects such as protruding jaws and huge eyebrows, heart problems and even cancer.

Partly because we only issue prescriptions in recommended doses, since the late 1990s we've never seen any such symptoms in our patients. Many people who publicly criticize HGH or tell their patients to avoid the hormone are endocrinologists, experts in allopathic medicine who specialize in the body's secretions of hormones.

From our view, these physicians are flat-out wrong when they lambaste injectable HGH. Endocrinologists either openly or unwittingly create many negative perceptions about using the hormone. They use these negative and fear-mongering comments as integral weapons in turf wars among various medical professions. Most endocrinologists want the positive attributes of HGH kept quiet, dropped under under the proverbial radar screen.

For the most part, endocrinologists learn the anti-HGH propaganda while in medical school. Then, following three years of intense training in internal medicine, in order to enter their eventual specialty as certified endocrinologists, these doctors must undergo an additional two or three years in fellowship training. In short, these sub-specialists want anti-aging medicine kept strictly in their domain.

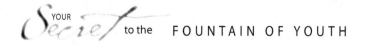

The turf wars intensify

By the time they finish their formal studies, many endocrinologists feel protective of what they've learned—jealous of any other professionals who would dare to claim expertise on the negatives or positives of HGH.

Meanwhile, endocrinologists steadily see an increasing number of other medical specialists who are seeking to prescribe HGH for the first time. They range from internists to gynecologists and sports medicine doctors, to retired psychiatrists.

Some professionals outside the practice of endocrinology get lured by the potentially lucrative business of prescribing HGH, as word spreads about its many proven benefits.

With greater intensity, we've seen a steady increase in head-butting among these various groups. These turf wars have been underway nearly 20 years, since the issuing of HGH prescriptions started kicking into gear in the late 1980s and early 1990s.

Feeling threatened, endocrinologists joined or solidified their associations with medical-related organizations or the federal government. These nay-sayers—some of them federal bureaucrats closely tied to endocrinologists and others within allopathic medicine—began pumping out false propaganda. They incorrectly claimed that anyone who prescribes HGH as a treatment for low levels of the hormone is practicing bad medicine.

Inconsistent prescription rules

As these disputes began reaching a boiling point, endocrinologists, Big Pharma, pharmaceutical lobbyists and their allies within the federal government conspired to impose stricter rules on the prescribing of HGH—when compared to criteria or protocol mandated for administering other hormones.

From the 1970s to the present day, standard allopathic doctors and endocrinologists have steadily and regularly increased the rate of prescriptions for such hormones as estrogen. We're unaware of any doctor being successfully sued for malpractice for putting a menopausal woman on that hormone. Under federal guidelines, physicians have the option of prescribing estrogen as replacement therapy.

Any suit would be considered weak against a physician for failing to prescribe to mature females the natural sex-related hormones estrogen, progesterone and testosterone. Likewise, the same physician could have a formidable legal fight in battling any attempts to sue for failing to prescribe to men the male hormone testosterone during andropause, the male version of menopause.

Yet paradoxically, if a menopausal woman suffers hypothyroid disease—symptoms suffered by 20-30 percent of women during this stage of life—and the physician fails to prescribe replacement thyroid hormones as therapy, that doctor faces a potentially successful legal suit.

Herein rests the stigma that endocrinologists, Big Pharma and the federal government have imposed on HGH, when considered as a treatment for somatopause, the body's natural lowering of growth hormone production.

In fact, HGH remains illegal to prescribe specifically and directly as a replacement hormone, the way estrogen is distributed in pharmacies. This makes absolutely no sense to us or to many others in anti-aging medicine.

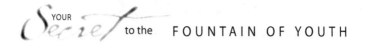

The feds tripped themselves up

In his opening statement at my trial, the prosecutor aimed a gun at his own foot by essentially telling the jury that: "Doctor Forsythe treats aging, and we all grow old and die. Why treat aging?"

This lame-brained statement told me loud and clear right away that we were going to win. I knew in that instant that the prosecutor was far behind the curve in advancements in modern science. To this point, backed by endocrinologists, Big Pharma and its political lobbyists, the federal government has considered using HGH for anti-aging as some form of quackery.

As my legal team expected, due to the prosecutor's extreme lack of knowledge, the innocent verdict set good case precedence. The jury's just and sound innocent verdict proved that doctors can give HGH as hormone replacement therapy, when practicing good medicine by properly testing and monitoring patients.

In seeking prosecution, the federal government had taken a very narrow view of what modern medicine is all about. They unsuccessfully tried to button-hole me as merely a physician who prescribes HGH, presumably the only treatment given by my office for anti-aging. In reality, though, I prescribe a wide range of bio-identical hormones, while also urging mature patients to eat proper foods and to exercise in moderation.

Certainly, the innocent verdict must have sent chills down the spines of endocrinologists who wanted to see me rot in jail, robbing the public of its ability to legally obtain HGH.

Shooting down objections

As medical professionals, the general rationale of the feds and endocrinologists for discounting the benefits of HGH strike us as mind-blowing. On a daily basis, we see many positive benefits, and negligible negative results that patients could easily overcome. And we fail to understand the motivation for their arguments, other than as a jealous attempt to establish turf control. These physicians want to prevent other doctors from encroaching on their professional territory.

Clinical results enable us to shoot down and obliterate all primary point-by-point statements that endocrinologists use in their fear-mongering tactics that stress the need to avoid objectionable HGH. Some of these bogus claims even got entered into the notorious Mitchell Report, an official congressional document on the use of steroids and HGH in professional sports. Among the primary issues:

Cancer

- **Fear-mongers:** People who use injectable HGH suffer a higher instance of cancers. The resulting disease riddles the body, resulting in a sharp decrease in life expectancy.

- **The facts:** When taken in proper doses of no greater than the maximum allowed, injectable HGH in mature people results in no increase in cancers. As an oncology practice, within our separate alternative medicine division, we would never consider giving HGH to mature people if injectable forms of the hormone had a slight chance of causing cancer. Children naturally have a lower incidence of cancers than mature people who have lower HGH levels. Although studies still need to be done, there's a real possibility that HGH may lower the rate of cancer in the mature. HGH improves immune function, which in turn lowers the risk of cancer.

Meantime, some studies indicate the incidence of prostate cancer might actually be lower among men taking injectable HGH. In general, there is an inverse relationship between higher rates of cancer and lower levels of HGH in the body. Also, children on HGH have not shown higher levels of cancer.

Acromegaly

- **Fear-mongers:** HGH causes acromegaly, particularly the enlargement of the brow, jaw, hands and feet. These characteristics could make a person look grotesque. HGH could cause excessive growth, perhaps up to 8 feet, resulting in severe health problems including heart disease and early death from an enlarged heart.

- **The facts:** Gigantism only occurs in children who have not experienced full bone growth. Symptoms of agromegaly would emerge only in extremely excessive doses. When taking HGH at proper levels, mature people experience no such characteristics. Remember, the adult dose is only 14 percent of a child's dose.

Gigantism

- **Fear-mongers:** Mature people who use injectable HGH could grow excessively tall, perhaps up to 8 feet, resulting in severe health problems such as heart disease or early death.

- **The facts:** Mature people using HGH never grow excessively tall. One positive benefit might be the curtailing of the body's natural shrinking process that impacts most seniors due to osteoporosis. HGH increases bone density.

As part of the aging process, many people who were 6 feet 2 inches tall from their 20s through 40s discover during maturity that they're now around 5 feet 10. The spine compresses like an accordion, causing mature people to lose from three to seven inches of their former height.

Healthy people have seven vertebrae in their necks, 12 in the thoracic spine, and five in the lumbar spine. When and if each of the 24 vertebrae compress by just a quarter inch as part of the natural aging process, a person becomes up to six inches shorter. Remember, studies show that HGH increases bone density in mature people by 0.5 percent to 1.5 percent per year, thereby preventing or decreasing the likelihood of osteoporosis-related fractures.

Also, children of short stature or dwarfism who receive injectable HGH as a treatment often grow in height, but never to the point of becoming extremely tall. The doses mature people receive are only 14 percent of those administered to young people with short stature.

Diabetes

- **Fear-mongers:** The use of HGH promotes or causes diabetes and the resulting serious medical complications.

- **The facts:** When given in proper doses, HGH never results in diabetes. Insulin problems could occur only in instances where the hormone gets administered in excessive amounts greater than the recommended doses. Although studies still need to be done, we believe injectable HGH actually lowers the possibility of diabetes because—as shown by our clinical results on a consistent basis—the hormone reduces body fat, a major contributing factor in generating the disease.

Hypoglycemia

- **Fear-mongers:** Unlike people with diabetes, whose bodies fail to produce enough insulin, people with hypoglycemia produce too much of the substance—resulting in glucose levels that are too low. The fear-mongers claim that HGH forces the body to produce more insulin than necessary.

- **The facts:** These problems rarely happen in healthy children, and the same is true for mature HGH patients. We monitor their blood during regularly scheduled follow-up visits and would notice any increases in insulin levels, but that has never happens.

Carpal tunnel syndrome

- **Fear-mongers:** Injectable HGH causes carpal tunnel syndrome, with primary symptoms including over-growth of the wrist tendons, pinching the median nerve in the wrist and resulting in numbness in the middle fingers.

- **The facts:** Personally, we know of only one case where such symptoms occurred, and that happened when a physician administered the hormone to himself in excessive amounts. The symptoms subsided when he decreased the dosage to acceptable levels. If HGH universally caused carpal tunnel syndrome, all children would suffer from it. None of our mature patients receiving proper doses experience the symptoms.

Muscles

- **Fear-mongers:** People become too big or muscular, to the point of being grotesque.

- **The Facts:** While HGH consistently increases muscle density in the mature, when administered in proper amounts the muscles never becomes excessive. Retired baseball star Jose Conseco, an admitted HGH user, never complained of looking "too ripped."

Joints

- **Fear-mongers:** People suffer severe joint pain, since injectable HGH causes excessive and unnecessary growth throughout the body.

- **The facts:** None of our mature patients—who did not previously suffer from arthritis or other diseases of the joints—ever experience new problems in this area of their bodies. Anyone who complains of joint problems might be exceeding appropriate doses.

Extended bellies

- **Fear-mongers:** Bodybuilders who use HGH experience extended bellies, an unsightly physical condition.

- **The facts:** Many body builders apparently administer HGH in excessive amounts. Our patients never experience this.

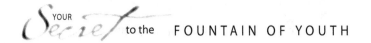

Pituitary tumors

- **Fear-mongers:** Tumors grow in or on the pituitary gland, cutting off or accelerating production of vital hormones including HGH and causing significant health problems.

- **The facts:** In our clinical research over many years, we've seen no sign whatsoever that injectable HGH administered in proper doses causes such tumors.

Summary

Various medical professionals stand to benefit from devaluing or criticizing HGH, amid turf wars concerning who controls distribution of this vital natural substance. Yet our clinical results consistently show that the legal prescribed use of the injectable form of the hormone is safe and effective when administered in acceptable doses.

CHAPTER 15

Wow, seniors! Enjoy physicial imtimacy!

Remember way back when you were a young adult, those years when you often enjoyed making love for hours on end? Perhaps you're among today's mature people who fondly recall what many of us refer to as the "after-glow."

If you've ever enjoyed fantastic sex as a young adult, you know the sensations. Many seniors fondly recall those days when immediately after orgasms, they felt as if all was one with the world—an overwhelming but calming sensation that if only for a brief moment they had somehow miraculously landed smack-dab in the center of a perfect universe.

Some of the world's most popular comedians joke that after sex, women often like to cuddle with their mates while many men find themselves dozing off. Endorphins that the body naturally creates due to physical stimulation can produce euphoric sensations that cause these behaviors.

These reactions, in turn, can help contribute to overall good health among young adults and even seniors who enjoy consistent, good and healthy sex. Orgasms aren't necessary each time, but certainly go a long way toward generating euphoria.

In many respects our bodies were made to procreate, to repopulate the Earth and to ensure the survival of our species. In fact, much of the physical and psychological makeup of humans is centered on one thing—having healthy physical intimacy and lots of it, too.

Why older people need sex

Human beings are considered the only mammal that can engage in orgasmic sex long after mature females in the population lose the ability to reproduce. But why does nature afford us this wonderful opportunity long after sexual intercourse loses any practical use, other than for physical pleasure?

A paradoxical situation emerges. Although physically capable of having and enjoying sex, many seniors find that over time their desire to copulate or to achieve orgasms wanes dramatically or ends altogether.

As to the question of why many seniors possess the capability of having and enjoying sex, some physicians and psychologists believe that nature wants us to bond with other humans as much as we want to throughout life. This, in turn, gives life itself some greater meaning for seniors, a motivation and purpose for sharing.

Yet when the libido decreases, mature people find themselves unwilling or incapable of even trying for sex—lacking motivation. Thus, nature in a sense gives dual signals: "You've got the tools to get laid, but you don't want to have that fun."

Certainly, drugs such as Viagra®, Levitra® and Cialis® have begun to correct erectile dysfunction, making sex among seniors more possible than before. Soon, increasing numbers of mature people will start getting amorous due to the growing popularity of injectable HGH spreads and bio-identical hormone replacement therapy

Craving physical contact

At present, science lacks an aphrodisiac pill that could suddenly turn older females and senior males into intimate moods. However, our laboratory results and conversations with patients clearly indicate that injectable HGH consistently turns the proverbial "I-want-sex" switch back into the "on" or "green light" position for seniors.

A large percentage of our older patients, both male and female, tell us that they gradually begin to crave and even yearn for sex—in many instances for the first time in decades. Just as they did as young adults, some of these delighted patients awaken refreshed in the morning, thinking about sex and asking themselves, "How am I going to get more of it?"

While masturbation emerges as an easy option or a quick fix for some, they know that the greatest pleasures usually derive from physical contact with another person. This, in turn, inspires the motivation necessary to generate relationships, which make life seem fuller and more delightful.

Have you ever known a senior who became isolated or lonely? Perhaps you or your mature parents stay at home just about all the time watching TV alone, or avoid in-depth conversations with people you meet on an everyday basis. Well, injectable HGH might help motivate such seniors to change such static behavior.

Just how amorous will you get?

While our tests have not been comprehensive to this point on HGH's impact on the libido, we find that overall these patients report a higher sex drive. Many physicians or pharmaceutical companies like to say in such instances that "individual results vary."

What's most important from the viewpoint of our patients, though, is that their physical desire clicks back into full gear or at least into a cruising mode. One patient might report a minimal or insignificant increase in libido, while another begins craving sex like a young adult.

Overall, although we have not yet formally charted these results, we can say with a fairly high degree of certainty that men and women have similar results overall—at least when it comes to regaining physical desire.

For many people, both young and mature, there's a need to look or at least seem physically attractive in order to become amorous. Perhaps due to the high attention our media plays on a youthful appearance, many patients—especially women—hold a need to look beautiful or at least alluring in order to crave intimacy.

The higher energy that results from taking injectable HGH can play a significant role in increasing such self-esteem, enabling those vital mating juices to flow once again.

Scream in ecstasy

In findings that might make the grandchildren of many seniors blush, in August 2007, the "New England Journal of Medicine" reported results of the first comprehensive survey on the sexual activities of people ages 57-85. The survey found that more than a fourth of those up to age 85 admitted to having sex at least once during the previous year.

These results show that many seniors can and want consensual sex, wiping out a long-held stereotype that sex is a fun activity reserved for the young.

As if these statistics weren't enough to stir the imagination, think of how these overall totals will increase once great numbers of seniors start using injectable HGH. Imagine the private screams of ecstasy that will reverberate within households of seniors across America.

The hit 1966 Broadway musical "Cabaret" made the phrase "money makes the world go round" popular worldwide. And in the same vernacular even today you could argue that "love makes the world go round" as well. While equating sex with love might raise some eyebrows, there's little doubt that enjoying more sex can generate lasting relationships and good health, particularly when practicing safe-sex methods.

Summary

Many seniors report a sharp rebound in their desire and sexual activity after beginning HGH regimens. For some mature people this development sparks a new zest for life.

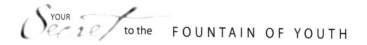

CHAPTER 16

The history of HGH law

During the late 1980s, amateur and professional athletes began obtaining manufactured HGH via illegal importation of the substance from Mexico, Canada and overseas. At the time, the federal Food and Drug Administration had not legally classified HGH, thereby never deciding whether the public could use the hormone as a drug or substance.

However, the agency continued empowering physicians to administer the hormone as a prescription drug, but only when doctors handled the patient's immediate care.

Sports trainers and team physicians told the FDA that athletes were using the substance. All along, the agency realized the difficulty involved in classifying HGH as a scheduled drug or a controlled substance.

To address this challenge, at the FDA's request in 1990 Congress augmented the original steroid law, inserting a provision making the use of HGH as an "anti-aging intervention" an illegal criminal act— punishable by up to five years in prison and fines up to $250,000. Yet at the time there were no anti-aging physicians in the United States.

Several years later the American Academy of Anti-Aging Medicine held its very first meeting. Dozens of physicians attended, rather than hundreds or thousands of doctors—totals that might have seemed appropriate consider the extensive public demand for HGH. By almost every account, of the physicians who attended, none knew that Congress had limited the use of HGH to very specific conditions. Meantime, a paradoxical situation arose, because the "Physicians Desk

Reference"™ or PDR, the publication used by physicians to review pharmaceuticals, states that any drug approved by the FDA can be used for off-label use. This means a physician can prescribe a drug for a purpose other than a specific type of condition that the substance is indicated to treat.

The government's ban against HGH for anti-aging, coupled with the ability of physicians to prescribe the hormone, resulted in a Catch-22 situation.

Worsening matters, the law basically tries to ignore that age-related growth deficiency syndrome is a proven scientific fact. A physician has an ethical duty to prescribe HGH, along with good medical care and testing, to each patient diagnosed with this condition.

At Life Extension Corporation, Steven B. Harris, M.D., says that HGH is the only pharmaceutical listed as illegal to prescribe for off-label use: "Even FDA-controlled substances, including narcotics, are legal to prescribe for off-label uses."

This paradoxical conflict has intensified a turf battle among many conventional board-certified endocrinologists and New Age "anti-aging" or "age management" physicians. The older, more rigid endocrinologists do not want family physicians, internal medicine physicians, gynecologists—and for that matter, any other specialist—encroaching on their territory.

Is this a pocketbook issue?

Stuck in a bind, some doctors continue prescribing the hormone. The "New England Journal of Medicine" reported in 2003 that one third of HGH prescriptions were for off-label uses.

Compounding the situation, the Internet blossomed into widespread public use in the mid- to late-1990s, well after Congress imposed the

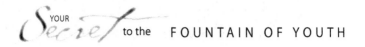

law. The World Wide Web enabled people in the U.S. to obtain HGH from international markets with greater efficiency.

The FDA has clamped down on the Internet-ordering market, requiring that only domestic doctors issue the hormone on an individual basis—and only to people under each physician's direct care. Ironically, the FDA's regulations specifying its own mission clearly states that the agency "does not regulate the practice of medicine."

In 2006, numerous physicians told "Forbes" magazine that thousands of physicians have been distributing HGH for anti-aging purposes, while the law banning the prescribing of the hormone for anti-aging purposes has rarely been enforced.

Some physicians today say during television interviews that injectable HGH causes diabetes and cancer, assumptions unsupported by allopathic medical literature. Even huge pharmaceutical manufacturers have told the FDA that to prevent misuse they tightly control distribution of the hormone to large medical centers and training hospitals.

In fact, primary care physicians and specialists in endocrinology, gynecology and geriatrics have been prescribing hormone replacement therapy for thyroid deficiencies, sex hormone deficiencies, and for adrenal gland inefficiency.

As a result, many physicians are asking, "Why is it illegal to prescribe—whether off-label or not—the use of human growth hormone for test-proven HGH deficiency syndrome?"

Among physicians indicating they're increasingly concerned, Dr. Harris says that "When your government determines for you, on penalty of long prison sentences, what is scientifically and medically correct—even on issues where reasonable, educated people disagree on the science—your society is in big trouble."

Responding to this dilemma, the American Academy of Anti-Aging Medicine assembled a legal team to protect physicians against untoward prosecution by state boards and federal regulatory agencies. The Academy strives to protect the rights of physicians to practice advanced preventative medicine for the benefit of patients.

"Aging is really a constellation of degenerative diseases or processes that lead to chronic disease and death," said Dr. Ronald Klatz, author of "Grow Young With HGH." Klatz acknowledges that physicians have yet to develop a way for us to avoid aging.

"You can, and doctors do every day, treat osteoarthritis, osteoporosis, Alzheimer's disease, macular degeneration and hormone replacement therapies, as well as heart disease and cancer," Klatz said. "By improving the quality of life and avoiding these diseases, you can live longer with improved functioning."

Most clinical physicians involved in anti-aging medicine agree that the hormone, when used properly in HGH-deficient adults, has numerous benefits on body composition, plus cardiac and cognitive function.

When considering all these various factors, any physician who fails to prescribe HGH where indicated would engage in unethical conduct and even malpractice. Such failure would be contrary to a patient's overall health and well-being.

"Given the state of scientific medical knowledge today, growth hormone is safe," said Ronald Rothenberg, M.D., author of a 2004 paper, "Anti-Aging Therapeutics," and a clinical professor of family medicine at the University of California at San Diego School of Medicine.

"Growth hormone replacement therapy is associated with decreased morbidity and mortality, less cardiovascular disease, less inflammation, improvements in body composition, improved exercise capacity, and a better quality of life," Dr. Harris said.

Setting off proverbial fireworks amid the discussion, the Oct. 26, 2006, issue of "Journal of the American Medical Association" stirred up huge controversy and discussion among anti-aging societies worldwide. The article criticized the routine use of HGH for anti-aging deficiencies.

"In my opinion the discussion is confusing and at times inaccurate," Dr. Ronald Rothenberg said later, in response to the article. "The article lumps together Web sites selling growth hormone illegally without medical supervision, over-the-counter products which may or may not contain growth hormone, and medically supervised treatment for adult-related human growth hormone deficiency syndrome.

"There has been extensive documentation in the peer-reviewed medical literature on the benefits and low-risk profile of growth hormone replacement therapy for age-related human growth deficiency syndrome."

Adding to the firepower, Dr. Klatz noted that the report also excluded patients who do not have HGH deficiencies. In addition, Dr. Allen Mintz, the director of Cenegenics Medical Institute in Las Vegas, one of the nation's largest anti-aging clinics, said an HGH-challenge test isn't required to prescribe the hormone for deficient adults.

"If physicians have a legitimate, clinically-based rationale for diagnosing a patient with HGH deficiency, the law does not restrict the physicians' judgment in this respect," Mintz said.

Summary

Sharp differences remain among various medical professionals on the legal and appropriate instances where physicians can prescribe injectable HGH. Even so, the "Physicians Desk Reference™" clearly states that doctors can prescribe any approved substance for off-label treatments. HGH falls within those parameters, since federal authorities classify the hormone as appropriate to use for certain medical conditions.

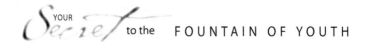

CHAPTER 17

Add Melatonin to your list of pharmaceuticals

We strongly recommend that people who use injectable HGH also take melatonin, a natural non-steroidal hormone available over the counter and an admirable performer in the anti-aging process. Russian studies have shown that melatonin replacement therapy expands the life spans of mice by up to 25 percent.

All along, however, pregnant or nursing mothers, or women trying to conceive, should avoid taking over-the-counter melatonin.

Clinical results consistently show that this hormone battles free radicals hidden in toxic substances from food, water and the environment that—if left unchecked—can contribute to the aging process. Melatonin also defends the brain function by warding off free radicals.

Just as impressive, even allopathic physicians know that melatonin may decrease heart disease and immune deficiency diseases. In a study at the University of Texas Health Center in San Antonio, rats given carcinogens before melatonin treatments had 50 percent less genetic damage than those without such therapy.

Often used to battle certain cancers, particularly of the prostate and breast, melatonin boosts the immune system while helping AIDS patients and people suffering from chronic depression. Researchers began studying melatonin in the 1950s. These professionals finally began realizing this hormone's many benefits in the late 1980s.

For many years airline personnel and frequent travelers have made melatonin a favorite, highly recommended treatment for jet lag. In animals, this natural substance controls seasonal rhythms such as migration, mating and even hibernation.

In nature, melatonin regulates the body's circadian rhythm, the daily 24-hour cycle that mandates vital functions. Besides behavioral processes, these include biochemical and physiological processes in animals, plants, fungi and certain bacteria.

Within humans, the small pineal gland the size of a date pit and shaped like a tiny pine cone at the center of the brain produces melatonin. The famed 17th Century philosopher Descartes called this gland "the seed of the soul." Surrounded by a rich blood supply, the pineal gland contains 100 times more serotonin than any other brain tissue.

An essential neurotransmitter, serotonin serves as an important precursor or direct parent of melatonin. Neurotransmitters play an essential role in modulating, relaying and amplifying signals between neurons and other cells.

The daily circadian rhythms regulated and controlled by melatonin include the secretion of HGH. Melatonin also regulates the secretion of the stress-regulator cortisol and the sex hormone testosterone, which manages energy, libido and red blood cell production—while also protecting the body against osteoporosis.

In addition, melatonin stimulates the pituitary gland's production of HGH, which—as stated earlier—peaks during REM or rapid eye movement sleep. Unless a person takes injectable HGH and over-the-counter melatonin, all these processes go haywire during the aging process.

Like HGH, the body's production of melatonin decreases as people age. Melatonin levels peak from ages 15-25, before decreasing to 15-20 percent of those levels by age 70. The problem becomes more complex because serotonin levels remain high in mature people. As a result, the balance between melatonin and serotonin weighs in favor of serotonin as we age.

Among mature people, a variety of negative symptoms can emerge, most notably interrupted sleep patterns, central sleep apnea, sexual dysfunction, depression and a tendency to develop Type II diabetes mellitus.

The eventual dominance of serotonin in mature people emerges as a harmful development, largely because melatonin plays a vital role in enhancing the essential sleep process, important to the body's healing. Remember that physicians know a good night's sleep serves as nature's best healing medicine. Most heart attacks occur in the early morning hours. Also, women are most likely to go into labor early in the morning.

Melatonin plays a role in many body functions

Physicians find little surprise when concluding that mature people who never take over-the-counter melatonin have decreased quality and duration of sleep, while immune functions, vitality and longevity diminish as well.

On the positive side, we know that eating fewer calories can increase the body's natural melatonin production. The essential amino acid tryptophan from food enables the body to create serotonin, which in turn gets converted to melatonin.

Thanks to the pineal gland's strategic location within the brain, the body secrets melatonin directly into the cerebrospinal fluid and the general circulatory system. However, the body markedly reduces the production of melatonin during daylight hours, following its usual peak at about 3 o'clock in the morning.

Medical professionals say that melatonin acts as the body's biological clock, due to the hormone's relationship to light and dark cycles. Seasonal changes impact this process, when daylight hours expand during summers and shorten during winters.

These biological changes cause fluctuations in the secretions of HGH, the stress-regulator cortisol and major sex hormones. Almost as if a nighttime burglar, melatonin seemingly comes alive during the dark when performing its work, before fading at the light of day.

Many medical professionals call melatonin a "third eye" because of its ability to control this daily cycling in mammals throughout the animal kingdom.

Follow a dosing pattern when starting melatonin

People older than 50 who use melatonin should start such regimens by taking lower doses, such as 1-3 milligrams at bedtime. This early process usually entails taking melatonin every other day or a maximum 5-6 days per week. Be sure to avoid taking over-the-counter melatonin at least one day per week, in order to allow the pineal gland to continue making this hormone uninhibited.

Later, after initial regimens have progressed awhile, some individuals can easily tolerate nightly bedtime melatonin doses of 10-30 milligrams.

Such high doses might become necessary in mitigating the negative impacts of sleep apnea. A disorder marked by potentially dangerous pauses in breathing while asleep, sleep apnea affects up to 20 percent of people older than 50. Physicians have been unable to find or develop an effective prescription drug to treat this condition. In higher doses as much as 10 or 20 milligrams taken before bedtime, melatonin may lesson the negative affects of sleep apnea.

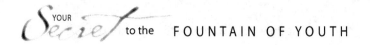

Summary

Hailed by many people as a wonder drug, melatonin should be taken in conjunction with HGH, thanks to its many health benefits ranging from the treatment of sleep apnea and immune deficiencies to possible increases in lifespan.

CHAPTER 18

More hormone replacement therapies benefit women

Along with using injectable HGH, women in their mid-50s and older can enjoy additional benefits by also using replacement therapies for other hormones. Women who employ these additional therapies often benefit from increases in muscle mass, decreases in body fat and increased energy, plus better mental function, and improved immune systems. Benefits in cholesterol levels and bone density often occur as well.

Other than HGH, the most common bio-identical hormone replacement therapies for women involve:

- **Estrogen**: A naturally occurring steroid, estrogen serves as the main female sex hormone primarily produced within the ovaries—and by the breasts, liver and adrenal glands. Estrogen performs an essential role regulating menstrual cycles and in developing secondary female sex characteristics such as breasts. Besides regulating height, estrogen plays an essential role in accelerating the metabolism to burn fat and increase bone density.
- **Progesterone**: The female menstrual cycle, pregnancy and the formation of embryos are regulated by this steroid hormone. Progesterone is primarily produced by the ovaries or gonads, the brain and also the placenta during pregnancy. Also in nature, yams are the primary foods that generate progesterone.
- **Testosterone**: The well-being and health of a person hinges largely on this steroid hormone produced by the male testes and female ovaries. While protecting against osteoporosis, testosterone increases red blood cell production and enhances the libido while increasing energy. Adult men produce 40-60

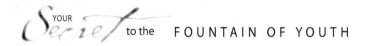

times more testosterone than women, but females show greater sensitivity than males to this hormone on a behavioral level.

To varying degrees, the levels of estrogen, progesterone and testosterone decrease in women as they age. In addition, individual women respond at different levels to bio-identical replacement therapy or BHRT. Every woman has a different level of absorption and varying degrees of metabolism.

Some controversies have arisen involving the use of bio-identical replacement therapy, particularly estrogen when applied as a cream. We say an emphatic "no" to people who ask if such therapy in the form of estrogen increases the rates of breast cancer and cardiovascular disease. We're pleased to tell patients that creams used in bio-identical replacement therapy are effective on all women.

Understand the impacts of the female life cycle

Hormonal imbalances occur in women before, during and after menopause, the period when a female's menstruation cycles ends. A bio-identical replacement therapy regimen can address a variety of adverse physical symptoms that women sustain during each of these life phases.

Besides heart palpitations, racing hearts and moodiness or mood swings, these symptoms can include erratic behavior or irritability, tender breasts, diminished sex drive and pain during intercourse due to vaginal dryness.

Compounding these problems, during the perimenopausal period just before, during and after menopause, some women also experience frequent urination, excessive weight gain, frequent vaginal yeast infections and diminished bone density.
As if all these problems weren't already enough, many maturing women complain of decreased energy or vitality, memory loss, joint

and muscle aches, lightheadedness, insomnia, hot flashes and cold or clammy skin.

Created from plant products in a bio-engineering process, bio-identical estrogen and progesterone hormones can be used to help battle these problems.

In addition to these bio-engineered hormones produced in laboratories, some medical professionals also recommend using synthetic hormones or the hormones from pregnant horses as supplements. However, synthetic hormones and hormones from mares fail to work as well as bio-identical products in the human female body.

Premarin™, a compound drug derived from the urine of pregnant mares, contains three forms of estrogen that naturally occur in human females; another 47 forms of estrogen from the urine never occur naturally within women.

Big Pharma avoids distributing such hormones

Similar to what happens with HGH and nutrients such as Vitamin C, large drug companies avoid distributing or actively marketing natural hormones through pharmacies—at least in large quantities. These firms lack the ability to patent and profit substantially from naturally occurring substances like hormones.

In 2002, the Women's Health Initiative studied hormonal replacement therapy on women before, during and after menopause. The study focused on Prempro™, a combination of two synthetic female estrogen hormones—Premarin™ from mares' urine, and Provera™, a progesterone.

Premarin™ had 10-15 percent of estriol that naturally occurs in human females, serving as the main protective estrogen in women. By comparison, bio-identical estrogen produced in laboratories contains 60-80 percent of the level of estriol that naturally occurs in adult human females.

In addition, Prempro™ contains only 5-15 percent of estradiol sex hormone, compared to bio-engineered products that contain 20 percent of the levels of this naturally occurring estrogen that women have. Also, Prempro™ contains 75-80 percent of the levels of estrone that this naturally occurring but potentially dangerous estrogenic hormone occurs in women.

The Women's Health initiative stopped its study of 16,000 women taking Prempro™ earlier than scheduled, citing results that showed severe risks of taking the product.

Among the findings: a 20 percent increased risk of breast cancer among all women in the study; a 20 percent increased risk of coronary artery disease of women in the study compared to control groups; a 41 percent increase in strokes; and a 111 percent increase in the risk of blood clots in the lower body.

Although these products remain on the market, some physicians avoid prescribing Premarin™ and Provera™, given their known risks.

By contrast, we're unaware of any studies revealing negative results involving bio-identical hormones intended to benefit mature women.

Topical creams also benefit women

Mature women also can benefit from a variety of topical creams developed as vital treatments within bio-identical hormone replacement therapy regimens. Compounding pharmacies create many of these creams by using natural foods or substances like soy or yam roots. Medical professionals prepare these substances, making exact replicas of female hormones that women's bodies naturally produce.

Using topical creams, estrogen replacement therapy can effectively diminish acne, facial hair, hot flashes, depression and joint or muscle pain. Meantime, these same treatments often increase breast fullness, nipple sensitivity, bladder control, vaginal lubrication, the intensity of orgasms and the clitoris' size and sensitivity. Female patients also enjoy improved sleep, better mental function and increases in bone mineral density.

Women also enjoy some of these benefits from low-dose bio-identical testosterone applied via bio-identical creams. Besides increases in energy, strength, bone density and libido, these changes include decreases in moodiness, depression and panic attacks.

Adding even more substantial benefits to these therapies, natural progesterone applied as bio-identical replacement therapy in the form of topical cream has many benefits as well. These include increases in appetite, fertility, and bone mineral density—plus decreases in premenstrual symptoms, mood swings, anxiety and depression. And less tissue growth occurs within or outside the uterus.

To their credit, since the mid-1900s, gynecologists, homeopaths and naturopaths have prescribed bio-identical hormone replacement therapies to mature women. But amazingly, despite the many benefits that maturing women receive from bio-identical replacement therapy, many allopathic medical physicians still refuse to issue such prescriptions.

Some medical professionals worry about the effects of too much or too little estrogen. Among potential negative outcomes in these situations:

- **Too much estrogen**: Fluid retention, oily skin, overly tender breasts, bloating, overactive libido and sexual aggressiveness, and increased sedation.
- **Too little estrogen**: Except for the libido, any or all the potential problems from having too much estrogen, plus increased moodiness and insomnia, plus a decrease in sex drive.

Understand the various application methods

Medical professionals use various methods and doses when applying estrogen, progesterone and testosterone in bio-identical replacement therapy. As a result, patients should understand the basics of applying each type of hormone. Among application methods for each:

- **Progesterone**: Partly because this medication will help you sleep, take at bedtime as either a cream or capsule. Never apply creams to fatty areas of the skin. Rubbing thoroughly at least 10 times, apply creams to clean, dry skin at the inner forearms, upper chest and neck, where the body can easily absorb the hormone. The cream usually dries within 5-10 minutes. Wait at least two hours to wash these areas, and avoid bathing, swimming or exercising during this period. Unless directed otherwise by a medical staff, women still in the menstrual phase should take progesterone creams or capsules on days 14-28 of their cycles. Because homeopaths consider daily applications of progesterone as safe, they sometimes issue full one-month supplies.
- **Estrogen**: The application of estrogen usually involves estriol, sometimes referred to as E-3, and the estradiol sex hormone, sometimes called E-2. Patients should apply estrogen-based creams the same way such ointments are administered for progesterone. Women still experiencing menstruation should take estrogen creams on days 1-15 of their cycles. Some patients wonder why estrogen applications are applied via creams rather than capsules taken orally. The liver and digestive tract

would rarely absorb the integral properties of estrogen when taken in capsule form.

- **Testosterone**: When applied as a cream, women should usually take this in the morning, preferably at the inner thighs, or behind the knees or lower legs. These creams can increase hair growth in areas where applied. So, some women prefer to administer these treatments to areas where they normally shave. Just like with progesterone, avoid applying to fatty areas of the skin. Use all application and cleaning methods necessary with progesterone or estrogen creams. Unlike creams and progesterone and estrogen, those with testosterone can be used daily.

Diet and exercise also play key roles for women

Professionals in anti-aging medicine emphasize diet and exercise play key roles, enhancing the overall quality of life and health in maturing women. Homeopaths and allopathic physicians urge these individuals to engage in both aerobic and anaerobic exercise, pilates and yoga. The general attributes of these types of activities are:

- **Aerobic exercise**: This involves a warm-up period, followed by a minimum 20 minutes of moderate or low-intensity exercise.
- **Anaerobic exercise**: These activities generally involve high-intensity activities such as cycling, running, swimming and strength training for short periods.
- **Pilates**: Developed by Joseph Pilates of Germany, this physical fitness regimen focuses on the body's postural muscles including the spine as deep torso muscles strengthen.
- **Yoga**: Created in India, offering various related mental and physical disciplines or philosophies, practitioners usually strive to control their bodies—while striving to achieve a variety of goals from better health to losing a sense of self.

Before beginning any exercise program, you should first consult your allopathic physician or homeopath to determine if you're healthy enough for such activity.

Just as important as exercise, the diets of maturing women near, during or after menopause should include organic fruits, healthy fats such as olive oil, and fish or poultry. Women also should strive to eat healthy carbohydrates in the form of vegetables and whole grains rather than from sugar, bread or pasta. Also, the principles outlined in three primary food-selection programs are highly desirable:

- **Zone Diet**: Developed by biochemist Barry Sears, this food-selection program entails comprising your diet of 40 percent carbohydrates, 30 percent proteins and 30 percent fats. Various studies indicate these ratios result in reasonable rates of weight loss.
- **South Beach Diet**: Dietician Marie Almon and cardiologist Arthur Agatston developed this diet or food-selection plan, heralded to low-fat diets developed in the early 1980s that the American Heart Association advocates. This diet essentially involves replacing "bad" fats and carbohydrates with their good counterparts. Rather than grains and sugars that are heavily refined, this diet favors whole grains, beans and vegetables that are relatively unprocessed. Meantime, saturated fats replace trans-fats.
- **Modified Atkin's Diet**: Developed by the late Dr. Robert Atkins, this low-carbohydrate food-selection system or diet—also low in saturated fat—attempts to make the body's metabolism burn stored body fat rather than burning glucose.

Summary

Bio-identical hormone replacement therapy provides numerous definite, predictable benefits to maturing women—improving their physical and mental health. Treatments that add or replace estrogen, progesterone and testosterone can emerge as vital enhancements to the many benefits of using injectable HGH, the "master hormone." Adding proper foods and exercise to these regimens improves overall health even more.

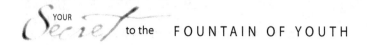

CHAPTER 19

Professional Sports: Our government tries to smash HGH

In his best-selling books "Juiced" in 2005 and "Vindicated" in 2007, former professional baseball player Jose Conseco opened the lid on the clandestine use of HGH and steroids in that sport. Conseco estimated that during the previous 20 years, up to 80 percent of pro baseball players had used performance enhancing drugs including HGH.

Once heralded as professional baseball's golden boy, a former Player of the Year and an ex-Most Valuable Player, Conseco earned two World Series rings. Coaches, players, teams and the news media ostracized and black-balled Conseco following the release of his first book, labeling the athlete as a "has-been." Many people called him a jealous retiree with a chip on his shoulder, concocting lies about his former teammates.

The controversy intensified when the 2006 tell-all bestseller "Game of Shadows" by Mark Fainarue-Wada and Lance Williams alleged that former San Francisco Giants baseball star Barry Bonds used performance enhancing drugs.

"Game" contends that former player Mark McGwire's record-setting 70 home runs in a single season in 1998—smashing the former records of Babe Ruth and Roger Maris—motivated Bonds to use such substances. Fainarue-Wada and Williams claimed that Bonds began using performance enhancing drugs including HGH via his relationship with the Bay Area Laboratory Co-operative.

In 2001, Bonds smashed 73 homers, a new single-season record. Yet the star power of this slugger who subsequently became a free agent diminished in the eyes of many when the "Game" book was released, perhaps inspiring authorities to step up a criminal investigation of his activities. In November 2007, a federal grand jury indicted Bonds on perjury and obstruction of justice charges, alleging that the athlete lied under oath about his use of steroids.

In 2002, Major League Baseball had launched a joint drug prevention and treatment program to look into the players' use of performance enhancing substances. Largely as a result of these findings, in 2005 the sport added HGH and 17 steroidal hormones to its list of prohibited substances.

Also in 2005, McGwire refused to answer questions under oath at a congressional hearing on steroids. In what some analysts attributed to McGwire's refusal to testify, despite his many various hitting records, he failed to get enough votes in 2007 and 2008 for induction into the Baseball Hall of Fame.

Earlier, as the controversy continued to swell, in March 2006 Major League Baseball Commissioner Allan "Bud" Selig asked retired former U.S. Senator George J. Mitchell of Maine to investigate allegations that the sport's players illegally used steroids and other performance enhancing substances.

During the next 20 months, investigators interviewed more than 700 people, including at least 500 current or former team employees, team physicians, athletic trainers and security agents. Officials attempted to contact 500 former players, but only 68 consented to interviews.

Issued in December 2007, the 409-page Mitchell Report, along with Senate hearings before it, left several athletes falling from grace, while vindicating Conseco's earlier allegations.

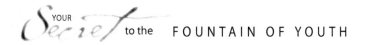

The controversial use of HGH in sports

The federal government and owners of major sports franchises should continue to develop and impose stringent bans of HGH among professional athletes. We strongly believe that competitors who abuse this natural substance to enhance their performance should face suspension or even expulsion from their jobs.

However, we also argue that professional athletes should be allowed permission to use HGH to rapidly accelerate the time needed to heal from injuries. Team owners, the fans and competitors deserve to have the most talented A-list athletes on the playing field or court rather than B-list or C-list team members that fewer people want to see.

Team owners make huge investments in their most popular players, sometimes tens of millions of dollars, attracting and keeping the best athletes. Fans that pay big bucks for season tickets in advance want and deserve the most talented competitors. And major advertisers want healthy athletes who are paid for endorsements.

The abuse of performance enhancing drugs by Major League Baseball players as far back as the 1980s contributed to the costly delay in allowing HGH to be accepted by the federal government and by a majority of allopathic physicians as replacement therapy for age-related deficiency syndrome.

The controversial Report did a horrible disservice to the public. Perhaps to scare teens and young adults from using HGH, the document exaggerated or flat-out gave wrong information about alleged health problems caused by the hormone.

We're amazed that when conducting research for the Report, its panel interviewed hundreds of people including baseball owners, athletic trainers, athletes and clubhouse employees—but only a handful of medical professionals, none of them homeopaths from highly knowledgeable clinics such as ours.

Adding to the public's misconception, the Report incorrectly stated that HGH has never been approved for cosmetic purposes or for anti-aging medicine. Here, we stress that the practice of anti-aging medicine involves far more than HGH, but also a variety of complimentary allopathic and integrative therapies.

In yet another grossly incorrect statement, the Mitchell Report says that "having a prescription for HGH for these unauthorized purposes (such as anti-aging) is a violation of federal law." Yet the innocent verdict in the government's criminal prosecution of me clearly and emphatically indicates otherwise.

Use HGH for rapid healing

Remember, our studies and various reports by other medical professionals consistently show that HGH rapidly accelerates the healing process, even in young adults. Under our proposal, sports teams could treat their injured players with this substance when conforming to the following conditions or criteria:

- **Doses:** Use only appropriate doses within recommended guidelines, in order to prevent adverse side effects.

- **Restriction:** Treat players while in the non-active or injured reserve mode, away from competition.

- **End-time:** Stop giving HGH treatments immediately or shortly before a player resumes competition.

- **Supervision:** All treatment should be supervised or prescribed by a licensed medical professional.

By adhering to these basic criteria, professional sports can get its players back in action in healthy conditions much faster than would normally be expected, while avoiding any chance that HGH will significantly enhance their athletic performances.

When conducting interviews, investigators or lawmakers working on the Mitchell Report determined that players also used HGH to heal injuries.

Prior to the newest restrictions and bans on performance enhancing drugs in their sport, numerous Major League Baseball players explained that they chose HGH because physicians had difficulty detecting the hormone in blood, urine or drug tests. Since then, enhancements in 24-hour-long urine tests have improved the ability to detect the use of injectable forms of the hormone.

The Report also cited additional health risks associated with obtaining steroids or HGH from potentially nefarious compounding pharmacies in Third World countries or China, providing drugs of "unknown or questionable strength, source or contamination." Adding to concerns, officials noted that the sharing of needles in locker rooms could, in rare instances, result in infections, hepatitis-B, hepatitis-C or even the precursor to AIDS.

By implementing an approved manner of using HGH for healing injured athletes, while also imposing a strict ban on the substance in other circumstances within professional sports, officials would eliminate such health concerns—also efficiently monitoring players for any inappropriate use of the hormone.

Athletes face a difficult reality

Before and since the Mitchell Report, professional athletes have faced a quandary when considering whether to use HGH to enhance their performance. Among the three primary factors many ask themselves:

1. **Dilemma:** Should I compete without performance enhancing drugs, possibly losing my competitive edge against teammates or opposing athletes who have fewer scruples?

2. **Leave:** Should I abandon my sport altogether, unwilling to use performance enhancing drugs that would put me on par with athletes who use them?

3. **Join:** Is it the best decision to start using these substances, largely in order to stay in my high-paid profession where people at this level have relatively short careers anyway?

As noted by the Mitchell Report, players who avoid steroids and HGH have "long complained that their teammates using steroids were taking their place on the starting roster." Taking this a step further, the Report also noted that the illegal use of performance enhancing drugs in Major League Baseball "victimizes the majority of players who do not use this substance."

Compounding the problem, as noted in the Mitchell Report, extortionists or gamblers—many with inside knowledge of which athletes take performance enhancing drugs—could seek to take advantage of the situation, sometimes via illegal bribery in hopes of rigging point spreads or game results.

Some lawmakers and investigators fear this could lead to poor performance and point shaving, plus an advantage in predicting game outcomes. Officials also worry that unscrupulous drug suppliers could dilute a drug or combine it with other substances, making a player dependent on the drug and its supply source.

By imposing the stringent ban on HGH and steroids, and implementing stringent testing, team owners sharply curtail these dilemmas and problems while keeping the playing field level for everyone. Just as important, the public should keep in mind that the legitimate and legal use of HGH for age-related human growth hormone deficiency syndrome has nothing to do with using this substance or steroids to enhance athletic performance.

Officials wrongly criticized HGH

When blasting HGH, the Mitchell Report largely cited complaints echoed by endocrinologists, whose fear-mongering assertions we already repudiated in a previous chapter.

Bogus symptoms of HGH citied by the report, which never occur when given in proper doses, range from acromegaly to enlarged flabby hearts. Other supposed symptoms that we've never seen include osteoporosis, thyroid disorders, and menstrual disorders.

Because the Report is loaded with misinformation on HGH, we urge Congress to create a special commission to investigate the erroneous and false conclusions about this vital and natural hormone.

By no means should the ban on HGH for the enhancement of athletic performance be construed as a strike against many clinically proven benefits, especially among mature people. Those who compiled the report are clearly off base when they claim that human growth hormone is a dangerous drug.

All along, we know that an athlete without an adequate medical background or lacking basic knowledge on administering HGH could double or triple the doses beyond the maximum-recommended limits. To their own detriment, some players might mistakenly believe that "if a little is good, more is better."

However, while doubling or tripling doses in clinical medicine causes severe side effects, especially when using substances like cortisone or androgenic steroids, the same cannot be said about HGH. This difference holds true even when users increase doses of the hormone two- or three-fold, usually without severe untoward symptoms.

Once again, allowing HGH for treatment of injuries while imposing stringent testing and restrictions among active players would sharply diminish such concerns.

Keep the ban on steroids

Remember that HGH is not a steroid. In contrast to HGH, which never causes severe health problems when administered in proper doses, steroids create or promote debilitating or life-threatening maladies from heart disease to cancer.

We've never heard of HGH causing life-threatening disease or death in any athlete. By contrast, many people have blamed anabolic steroids for causing the severe illnesses or premature deaths of athletes like former Oakland Raiders football player John Matuszak, who died in 1989 at age 38 from apparent heart problems. Whether any alleged use of steroids caused Matuszak's death remains speculation. According to news reports, his sister also died young due to heart problems, pointing to a possible genetic disorder.

In any case, we're certain that steroids can cause severe health problems, especially when mismanaged or given in improper doses. These dangers hold true among androgenic steroids that control masculine characteristics, and among cortical steroids that impact everything from motor skills to vision.

Besides promoting cancer, steroids can create a susceptibility to viral or bacterial infections, diabetes, obesity in the middle section of the body, and thin or gangly arms and legs.

Worsening matters, people who take steroids develop or suffer from weakened capillaries, making them bruise easily—even when lightly

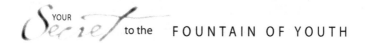

bumping into something such as a chair. These people often suffer stretch marks, stomach ulcers, and yeast infections in the mouth or vagina.

Severe weakness in the upper or lower extremities may occur. For people taking massive doses of steroids, everyday tasks like getting out of chairs become difficult.

A huge list of other potential maladies includes enlargement of the heart, congestive heart failure, glaucoma, thyroid disorders, hypertension, osteoporosis, menstrual irregularities, erectile dysfunction, and increases in bad cholesterol.

Adding to these woes, when given for performance enhancement, androgenic steroids or testosterone could cause increased aggressiveness or "roid rage," an unhealthy increase in red blood cell levels, testicular shrinkage, accelerated baldness, facial hair—a condition known as hirsutism—in females, facial or truncal acne, and a generalized increase in moodiness.

In our clinical opinion, all these various symptoms associated with steroids are never seen in patients receiving correct doses of HGH. Remember, the adult dose of HGH for age-related deficiency syndrome is an average one-seventh or 14 percent of the childhood dose. By extrapolation, HGH is seven times safer in an adult with a larger body than it is in children.

Summary

Many of our most cherished professional athletes have made serious mistakes in abusing steroids and HGH. Moving forward, we can turn these lessons to our advantage, improving the health of athletes by strictly banning the unauthorized use of HGH for performance enhancement, while also allowing injured athletes to use the hormone to promote a more rapid healing response.

CHAPTER 20

Conspiracy revealed: The politicians, allopathic physicians, Big Pharma & the media

An unholy matrimony thrives among the politicians, Big Pharma, the media and allopathic physicians as they work together to deny you the right to use injectable HGH. These primary problems work against the public interest:

- **Media:** Controlled by huge conglomerates that depend on significant advertising from Big Pharma, the news media fails to report in a bold and vibrant manner that HGH is helpful and appropriate for mature people when prescribed in proper doses. By reporting the accurate and indisputable facts you've learned here, a media outlet would stand to lose significant advertising revenues from Big Pharma, thereby cutting off a major potential revenue source for its parent company.

- **Politicians:** Largely influenced by huge campaign contributions from Big Pharma and by the industry's lobbyists, politicians have imposed stringent regulations that benefit these mega corporations—rather than the best interests of consumers.

- **Allopathic physicians:** Standard-practice doctors must comply with stringent regulations imposed by Big Pharma and the federal government, a process that—amazingly—involves the shunning of such natural substances as HGH and Vitamins C and D. While avoiding potential natural cures, these doctors prescribe drugs, some that collectively kill more than 300,000 patients per year.

- **Big Pharma:** Board members and top executives—including the presidents or chairmen of pharmaceutical companies— often earn tens of millions or even hundreds of millions of

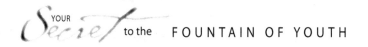
dollars per year. Their firms dole out incentives that motivate allopathic physicians to prescribe drugs, some potentially harmful. Many thousands of Big Pharma lobbyists work in Washington, D.C., urging Congress to ban the uses of natural substances like HGH, while endangering the public with potentially harmful drugs.

Working against the public interest, these bizarre professional relationships pose a real and dangerous conflict, resulting in an anti-trust atmosphere that promotes anti-competitiveness within segments of the medicine and food industries.

The fear-mongers would tell you that we're exaggerating in making these pointed negative statements. Yet these many unsavory relationships are well-documented, part of the public record—details laid out everywhere from the Congressional Quarterly to drug company stockholder reports.

Discover the drug companies' biggest problem

The drug companies dislike healthy natural substances like HGH and Vitamin C because those life-giving materials cannot get patented, preventing these items from getting sold by mega-pharmaceutical companies to the public at an exorbitant profit. Acting as an agent for Big Pharma, the federal government has produced, published and distributed various reports that strongly criticize natural materials that our bodies need for us to live.

Revealing itself as a pathetic agency in the pockets of Big Pharma, federal agencies strongly blasted high doses of Vitamin C, championed by Linus Pauling, the winner of the 1954 Nobel Prize in Chemistry for his pioneering work in the substance—which he personally used daily until dying in 1994 at age 93.

Worsening matters, federal researchers have consistently blasted a wide variety of natural substances. In the pockets of Big Pharma, the federal Food & Drug Administration often acts as if its federal bureaucrats have a better understanding of our bodies than does Mother Nature. This federal agency's lame-brained policies become especially offensive when HGH gets thrown into the mix.

Federal researchers and government agencies they work for have consistently issued allegations against natural substances, without mentioning the extremely dangerous drugs that the agency has approved. By some estimates, government-approved pharmaceuticals cause up to 300,000 deaths per year. Various rankings list prescribed drugs as among the sixth to the eighth leading cause of death.

By contrast, no one has ever died from Vitamin C or even HGH when prescribed and administered in proper doses. That's because our bodies yearn for such natural substances. Yet amazingly the federal government refuses to acknowledge that Vitamin C cures or lessens symptoms of scurvy, a disease caused by the lack of this substance, or even that HGH creates muscle mass and decreases body fat while providing a wide variety of other benefits.

What motivates the federal government?

Various vitamins can cure diseases, such as Vitamin B12, which treats the otherwise fatal pernicious anemia. However, the federal government states that anything that cures, mitigates or treats disease must be a pharmaceutical or drug rather than a natural substance.

As a result, many federal regulations fail to make common sense. This constitutes a sad state of affairs, since the agency wields huge influence on state medical boards, plus their combined organization, the Federation of State Medical Boards. Kissing up to the federal government, these boards seek out and punish any physician who thinks out of the box, who seeks to prescribe natural substances like HGH rather than high-cost drugs.

Federal and state officials label such medical professionals as "disruptive physicians," subject to censorship, fines or expulsion from the profession. Any doctor who refuses to strictly follow narrow guidelines set in the "Physicians Desk Reference™" on prescription drugs is refusing to follow straight-and-narrow criteria.

For instance, adding vitamins and minerals to standard chemotherapy treatment might be considered disruptive. Could these regulations stem from the fact that such a regimen would fail to depend solely on high-priced pharmaceuticals embraced by Big Pharma?

When HGH enters the mix, the oligarchy of Congress and Big Pharma become concerned since the hormone threatens numerous high-priced drugs—from weight loss pills to pain pills.

Were Big Pharma and allopathic physicians among my secret accusers?

At the time federal agents raided our practice, we had perhaps 12-20 patients taking prescribed HGH. By comparison, another Reno-area physician had at least 1,000 such patients and a local hospital even opened an anti-aging facility serving just as many people. So, why did the feds target us, rather than thousands of other physicians nationwide?

As stated earlier, perhaps we'll never know for sure. Our practice was small potatoes in the local market, insignificant on a national scale. Maybe investigators and prosecutors wanted to shut down effective alternative cancer-treatment protocols that I have developed. Under that scenario, my guess is that they failed to find any criminal activity, so they cooked up the bogus HGH charges in an attempt to shut us down.

Naturally, a new cancer treatment considered as a cure or at least highly effective in eliminating symptoms could cause huge, irreversible damage to Big Pharma. What better way to protect their own anti-competitive atmosphere than to shut me down.

To carry out their malicious, self-serving plan, during their investigation the feds violated the privacy of more than 220 of my patients—ordering me to duplicate these individuals' medical charts for prosecutors and for my defense attorneys. This forced me to violate the Hippocratic Oath, mandating that I violate my patients' privacy.

Were Big Pharma, politicians backed by its contributions, the industry's high-paid lobbyists, the media and allopathic physicians conspiring against me? Remember, numerous local news media outlets seized upon the story after my arrest and during the subsequent trial, attempting to ruin my professional reputation.

Many prominent people got caught into the mix

Whether the feds wanted it this way or not, many prominent people who were my patients got caught into this whirlpool. Some of the most prestigious officials in Nevada were swept up in the controversy, including prominent politicians who have great influence on the medical and pharmaceutical industries.

Rather than getting stuck on these complex details, suffice it to say here that, for the most part, the national media swept the arrest and subsequent trial under the proverbial rug. Could this have been because Big Pharma wanted me removed from the picture and made as an example, while these corporations strived to avoid any self-incrimination into its own selfish dealings?

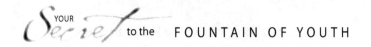

Summary

To the detriment of the public, an unholy alliance exists that has strangled the health and pocketbooks of consumers nationwide—a nefarious association among Big Pharma, the mainstream media, allopathic physicians, Congress and the federal government.

CHAPTER 21

The HGH protocol we wrote for the FDA: What it means to you

Protocol established major breakthrough for medicine

The jury's unanimous innocent verdict and the national protocol on HGH that I developed for the FDA established major, positive guidelines for the medical industry, expanding and solidifying instances where physicians can use this hormone for treatment.

Yet sadly, due to minimal publicity about this significant protocol, many doctors and medical professionals are either unaware that the document exists or they're afraid to embrace the protocol for fear of unjustified reprisals from the federal regulators.

Hopefully, widespread publicity about this book will teach and motivate doctors, after they learn that the protocol's objective was to expand on-label, medically necessary uses of growth hormone replacement therapy. As outlined by the protocol, the expanded uses are:

- **Aging:** Therapy for adults older than 40 with normally occurring decreases in HGH
- **Heart problems:** Treatment of congestive cardiomyopathies, or heart muscle diseases, and congestive heart failure
- **Burns:** Treatment of severe burn patients
- **Fatigue:** Treatment of chronic fatigue immune dysfunction syndrome or fibromyalgia
- **Heavy people:** Treatment of morbid obesity
- **Brain:** Treatment of traumatic brain and spinal injuries
- **Sports:** Treatment of professional sports injuries
- **Sleep:** Treatment of obstructive sleep apnea (OSA)

As noted earlier, until I submitted this protocol, the only established and approved therapies for HGH were for treatment of: AIDS wasting disease; short stature or dwarfism in children; and for short-bowel syndrome.

Mandatory medical history reviews

Under the protocol, when considering whether to implement growth hormone replacement therapy, physicians must continue to use standard and acceptable methods of discovering, reviewing or charting the complete and comprehensive medical histories of patients.

When considering HGH, this process involves a thorough examination that reviews or determines any history of documented hormonal deficiencies. This involves reviewing medical records to determine the prior use of hormone replacement therapies, and also checking the history of pituitary tumors, surgery, radiation therapy and trauma or prior chemotherapy.

Patients suffering from various pituitary deficiencies have an increased probability of having indications signaling a need for growth hormone replacement therapy.

Physicians also need to check for signs and symptoms consistent with HGH deficiencies, such as easy fatigue, a lack of energy, a decreased libido, poor exercise tolerance and sleep disturbances.

The protocol also tells doctors to look for contraindications, factors or conditions that increase the risks to patients who are being considered as candidates for growth hormone replacement therapy. These include patients with active cancer, Type 1 or Type 2 diabetes mellitus, carpal tunnel syndrome, and a variety of factors known as metabolic syndrome.

As with standard exams, each physician should use his or her medical judgment when ordering and subsequently reviewing medical tests. As stated in the protocol, "unfortunately, with growth hormone deficiency there is no single perfect and reliable test." Growth hormone has a short life of less than 20 minutes in the blood stream.

Review important medical considerations

The protocol notes that physicians consider many methods for the testing of HGH as impractical, largely because the hormone is primarily produced during rapid eye movement (REM) sleep—thereby making accurate hormone-detection methods impractical.

The protocol states that "short of this, the next most reliable and practical test is the liver metabolite of HGH called IGF-1." In addition, there are a number of cumbersome, risky or flawed tests that include the stimulation of HGH with arginine, clonidine, glucagon, L-dopa, insulin and propanolol.

Of these, the insulin tolerance test is thought to be the best predictor of growth hormone deficiency. Patients who fail to respond to insulin-induced hypoglycemia are likely to have a deficiency in growth hormones.

But this dangerous test carries all the risks of hypoglycemia including sweats, nausea, vomiting, mental aberrations, hypertension and possibly seizures. Also, physicians should avoid considering patients with coronary artery disease as candidates for the insulin stimulation tests.

In addition, clinicians should remain aware that poor nutrition, hepatic disease, severe diabetes mellitus and untreated hyperthyroidism can reduce IGF-1 levels. So far, attempts to measure IGF-binding proteins called IGFBP-3 have failed to achieve superior results when compared to conducting IGF-1 testing alone.

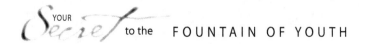

Our perseverance paid off

All these positive developments became possible thanks largely to the perseverance of my attorney, Kevin Mirch. As the scheduled fall jury trial approached, in August 2007 Mirch reached an agreement with the federal prosecuting attorney. At the time, from the view of my defense team, the prosecutors seemed to realize that I never even came close to committing a crime.

Working with Mirch, the prosecutor reached an agreement to have me write the official protocol on the use of HGH in age-related deficiency states, an official document for submission to the federal Food and Drug Administration. Under the government's initial proposal, I would have paid a $50,000 fine or settlement amount.

Taking this effort seriously, along with Mirch's wife, attorney Marie Mirch, our co-counsel, we embarked on a four-day fact-finding mission to Chicago for meetings with principals of the 20,000-member American Academy of Anti-Aging Medicine. These experts included some of the first physicians to prescribe HGH to mature adults.

After a careful, methodical, step-by-step review with these professionals, upon returning to Nevada I began writing the FDA's official protocol while following criteria and documentation approved or reviewed by some of my most prestigious peers.

On schedule and as promised, by late August 2007 I completed the document, which my attorneys submitted to prosecutors. Soon afterward, the federal attorneys told us that they had sent the document to the FDA in Washington, D.C., for further review.

Federal agency never responded

Although the FDA had officially requested that I create the protocol as part of a settlement agreement, the agency never sent us an answer.

Then, in early September 2007, the prosecuting attorney perjured himself at a pre-trial hearing, telling the judge that there had been no settlement agreement—when in fact a promise had been made, which we kept as our part of the bargain by developing the FDA's official protocol on HGH.

In discussions with Mirch, the prosecutor had previously agreed to wipe the slate clean of any criminal indictment—avoiding any negative impact on my medical license. Meantime, the prosecutor also had agreed to drop any investigation of me, without pursuing or filing misdemeanor or felony charges.

In a complete reversal of the government's position, the prosecutor falsely told the judge that there had been no settlement of any kind, and that I had agreed to be fined $50,000 and put on probation for 18 months—putting my medical license in jeopardy. Of course, we never even entertained such an agreement because I was innocent, coupled with the fact that such a settlement would have put my medical practice in an untenable position.

Like a guilty child caught with his hand in a cookie jar, the prosecutor clung to his new false story. As a result, because both legal teams presented different versions of what transpired, the judge decided to proceed to a jury trial.

From Mirch's view, Big Pharma, its lobbyists and politicians they support still wanted me punished for something I had never done, the bureaucrats embarrassed that I had developed the federal government's official HGH protocol.

We set legal precedence

In Mirch's view, the case established legal precedence thanks to the jury's verdict, plus the fact the FDA never responded or contacted us

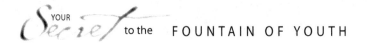

about the protocol document—without rejecting or commenting on the official publication that they asked me to develop.

Mirroring Big Pharma's persistent incompetence, through their own inept behavior the prosecutors cleared the way for landmark expansions in the legal, permissible and ethical uses of HGH.

To put it mildly, unskilled and heavy-handed federal tactics cleared the way for a ground-breaking expansion in the use of HGH, a positive C-change in medicine that hopefully will last for many generations. Physicians, government agencies and charities use the term "C-Change" in referring to their individual and collective efforts to manage or cure cancer.

Until this point, the federal government and allopathic physicians had not seriously considered the on-label use of HGH for serious, life-threatening medical conditions such as severe obesity or critical burns. Prior to the FDA's acceptance of my protocol, the on-label prescribing of HGH for such conditions was considered a criminal offense.

Summary

Thanks to what we personally consider bungling and inept federal prosecutors, we wrote a landmark protocol for the FDA that gives average citizens the ability to use injectable HGH when legally prescribed in safe amounts.

CHAPTER 22

Criminal trial sparked national ramifications

Needless to say, the conspiracy to convict me swelled to the point that the government committed a minimum 18 instances of malicious prosecution. Despite the federal attorneys' heated efforts, the entire power and might of our nation's government proved inept when pitted face-to-face with my legal team, Kevin and Marie Mirch.

Amid the trial, I kept wondering who had complained to the various federal agencies including the FBI. Remember, from our view, Earlene became a prime target due to her rising star power in the Republican Party.

Trying to shoot me down in the prime of my career, the various medical boards of allopathic physicians, Big Pharma and the politicians supported by the industry might have put me in their crosshairs—the conspirators distasteful of my alternative medicine practice. Where was justice, when I did not even know my true accuser?

Worsening matters, as we later discovered, the government had withheld "exculpatory evidence," a legal term referring to details that would have been favorable to me as a defendant, likely to result in an innocent verdict. Had prosecutors feared that their case was so weak that they felt a need for more trumped-up ammunition to win?

WARNING: Our government tells lies

Why had the government sought a fraudulent settlement agreement? And why did the prosecutor perjure himself to the judge by lying, saying essentially that "no settlement agreement had been reached"—

when in fact the document had been signed by this federal attorney, the judge, and my lawyer?

As if to add pain to an already-difficult situation, our clinic's disgruntled former employee—along with her husband—sat on the prosecution side during the trial. Was this the woman's perverted way of wanting to see me found guilty?

A vindictive former physician, who once rented space in my office, apparently tried unsuccessfully to tip the scales of justice by suddenly becoming a witness for the prosecution in grand jury hearings. I later saw this physician's affidavit that had been given to federal agents, basically stating that he disagreed with my use of HGH, when in fact this same doctor—himself—had practiced the same protocols.

Adding to the mystery, a different attorney other than the Mirches—a former long-time business lawyer that once represented Earlene and I—turned against us and our current legal team. The former attorney had attempted to quash our subpoenas of valuable witnesses, including a top Nevada official and a major media personality.

Before the trial began—but late in the information discovery process— the prosecution had continued to call and recruit my former patients in an attempt to get them to testify against me. Had prosecutors feared their weak case needed more ammunition to win?

Tears filled my eyes

At 8:30 in the morning on Nov. 1, 2007, I went to work as usual after the jury had deliberated less than a day. One hour later, members of my front office staff told me they had received an urgent message for me to go to the courthouse right away. I drove straight there, unaware at the time that Earlene had not received the message while in the shower at our home.

I stood with Kevin and Marie Mirch as the judge entered the courtroom, telling us that a verdict had been reached. Then, the jury marched into the courtroom, each panelist somber as I strived to discern any sign of the verdict from their body language.

For a fleeting moment after the foreman handed a written document stating the verdict to the judge, I briefly thought: "This must sincerely be a guilty verdict"—since on various TV shows security personnel are absent from courtrooms when an innocent verdict is read. By contrast, in this moment various officers or marshals stood watch.

The judge briefly looked at the document before handing it to the court recorder, who promptly read that the jury had reached a "not guilty" verdict. Marie, Kevin and I hugged each other. Tears welled up in my eyes and Kevin's; Marie refrained from crying, though I felt the emotion in her body.

For the most part, I felt pleased with the media response. However, the local newspaper refused to publish a correction that I had requested.

An article in a Las Vegas publication after the verdict quoted me as saying that while federal regulations are responsible for 250,000 deaths per year from approved drugs, they thought we would walk away from the agency's and the prosecutor's crude attempt at legal extortion.

The Nevada news media gave immediate coverage

The online "Health Freedom Alliance Newsletter" made it clear that the henchmen of Big Pharma had been "furious with federal prosecutor Brian Sullivan when they learned of the settlement agreement that he personally had negotiated with Dr. Forsythe." The emailed newsletter stated that Sullivan actually perjured himself in testimony.

And on the day of the verdict, the "Nevada Appeal" newspaper in Carson City, a 30-minute drive from Reno, quoted Kevin Mirch as saying, "You don't let an unqualified, sick person (the federal agent) make the decision to indict a doctor who has a sterling reputation for years and years and years."

Taking this a step further, nearly two weeks after the trial our law firm, Mirch & Mirch, issued a press release, quoting Kevin: "This was the most obscene miscarriage of justice I have witnessed and the jury agreed with us" after deliberating less than two hours.

The prosecution's effort had progressed under the watch of the U.S. Attorney for the District of Nevada, Daniel Bogden—eventually fired from the job, among controversial terminations of various U.S. attorneys nationwide by then-U.S. Attorney Alberto Gonzalez. Bogden subsequently testified before Congress, stating that the attempt to prosecute me had played a key role in his firing.

"The only reason the feds have been caught in this web of deceit is a brave and courageous doctor stood up and challenged their lies," Mirch said in the press release. "It's amazing what they did in their raid; how they broke the law during the investigation; how their case was so shabbily presented in court."

Physicians nationwide gave positive response

Homeopathic physicians nationwide gave a positive response, sending me cards and letters of kudos and encouragement. The trial's outcome tore down a curtain of fear. Some medical professionals had worried that a guilty verdict would end their ability to legally prescribe HGH, a core service in many of their practices.

Indeed, my arrest and trial had received little national coverage in the mainstream media at the time. That failed to curtail curious medical industry professionals, many who followed developments via the

Internet. I'll always remain grateful for their messages of support and encouragement.

Even more important, since early childhood in my mind all competent and God-fearing criminal prosecutors were representatives of a greater good, our public servants for fighting the wicked elements within society.

Yet this case taught us a serious lesson, as we learned that federal prosecutors can and do at times represent ill-intended forces, selfish or evil elements intent on circumventing the actions of good people in favor of greedy mega-corporations.

Summary

The government's unsuccessful attempt to prosecute me set a historic legal precedence, clearing the way for the public to use legally prescribed HGH for many generations to come.

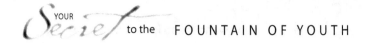

CHAPTER 23

Discover our controversial recommendations

Although prosecutors, with the blessing of the federal government, wanted to make a national example of me, these bureaucrats should suffer several legal consequences for their inept and selfish actions in attempting to keep the public from rightfully receiving legally prescribed HGH—pursuing my prosecution as part of their selfish plan.

We encourage the president of the United States, Congress, the FDA, administrators of various federal agencies and the mainstream media to implement the following procedures:

- **OFFICIAL REPORT:** Congress should hold hearings on the HGH issue and on the federal government's unholy matrimony with Big Pharma. Afterward, the panel should issue an in-depth report with full recommendations on how to cut back the influence of Big Pharma and to minimize its exorbitant drug prices. Officials should issue these findings with the same publicity that the widely reported Mitchell Report received.

When conducting its initial investigation, the panel should interview HGH experts such as us, plus numerous doctors of homeopathy nationwide. These experts should get equal emphasis during the investigation, just as much attention to any statements given by allopathic physicians or representatives of Big Pharma. All along, homeopathic physicians should be given a method to dispute any inaccurate statements made by Big Pharma and the so-called standard medical industry.

- **PROFESSIONAL SPORTS:** The panel should shoot down various misstatements made about HGH in the Mitchell Report, while recommending ways that this natural substance could and should be used for the appropriate treatment of sports injuries.

- **LEGALIZE HGH:** Congress should strengthen laws legalizing HGH, making it clear to the public that this substance is beneficial as an anti-aging treatment, never harmful when administered in proper doses. The FDA should fund and start a multi-year, multi-billion dollar advertising campaign, applauding the use of natural substances including legally prescribed HGH and vitamins.

In addition, the FDA should work with various state medical boards, ensuring that the laws on administering HGH are uniform from state to state—eliminating the confusion about certain professionals being able to issue HGH prescriptions in some jurisdictions but not in others.

- **THE FDA:** The federal agency should conduct, publish and distribute various intensive studies and reports, stating the many benefits of individual natural substances including HGH and vitamins—while refuting and discounting its own previous statements that natural substances are harmful to people.

- **ALLOPATHIC MEDICINE & HOMEOPATHY:** Congress should force the FDA to allow standard-medicine physicians to work alongside homeopaths or at least in the same office facilities. Such integrated treatment methods have been successful throughout Europe and China for centuries, and elsewhere in the world, but never in the United States where such associations are prohibited or discouraged due to the unsavory influence of Big Pharma.

- **PHARMACEUTICAL LOBBYISTS:** As noted earlier, many thousands of pharmaceutical industry lobbyists in Washington, D.C., work full-time to convince lawmakers to shut out homeopathic medicine in favor of Big Pharma and allopathic physicians, plus the high-priced drug prescriptions that they administer. Congress should work to curtail the influence of these lobbyists, while severely limiting or removing altogether the ability of such companies to contribute to political campaigns.

- **ACCOUNTABILITY:** Congress should impose stringent laws, making the executives of pharmaceutical companies accountable for the tens of thousands of deaths caused yearly by so-called legal prescription drugs. Remember, HGH and vitamins in appropriate amounts have never caused a single death. In our view, although it has never received adequate publicity, the damage Big Pharma has caused society rivals or far surpasses the Enron Scandal, which resulted in the imprisonment of several executives of a former electricity, natural gas, communications, pulp and paper company.

- **PROSECUTORS:** Federal officials and the U.S. Attorney should issue reprimands, possible dismissals and a statement of "no faith" against the prosecutors who maliciously attempted to convict me. These penalties should include substantial monetary fines and minimum three-year disbarment from law practice. This action should serve as a notice, putting other prosecutors on alert nationwide that the public and our government will not tolerate the abuse of the legal system, especially when wrongfully using it as a tool for Big Pharma.

- **ADVERTISING RESTRICTIONS:** Big Pharma should be allowed to continue advertising in print, radio, TV and on the Internet. However, in order to minimize the unfair influence these mega-corporations wield over the mainstream news media, the federal government should provide tax incentives to those companies when they also advertise the benefits of homeopathy and natural substances.

Summary

In the wake of my trial and its aftermath, our government, pharmaceutical companies and the general public should seize and benefit from this momentous opportunity to bring the many benefits of HGH and other natural substances to the general population.

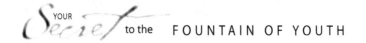

BONUS SECTION

CHAPTER 24

Discover how to become and remain youthful

With increasing frequency, scientists have begun announcing the good news that to a large extent they consider the aging process as preventable and treatable, rather than merely inevitable.

As we mature, for both genders our ability to appear and feel young involves more than merely human growth hormone replacement therapy. Exercise, food selections, hormonal supplements, minerals and vitamins play integral roles in this process. People who employ a balance of these factors position themselves for healthy, quality-filled aging—while lessening the possibility of chronic degenerative diseases like cancer.

Scientists and medical experts have yet to discover a single "magic potion" capable of preserving our youth. As already shown, injectable HGH can go a long way toward enabling us to recapture that vibrant, healthy aura enjoyed during our younger years. Just as important, certain natural foods provide many of the so-called amazing ingredients likely to slow or even reverse the impact that the passing decades took on our bodies.

Keep in mind from the start of this process that the food we eat hails as the most important factor in the body's underlying health and well-being. Proper exercise and adequate sleep go a long way toward eliminating stress or anxiety, unwanted factors in causing the body to age faster than desired. Some physicians consider aging as a disease brought on by poor or inadequate dietary choices.

Despite advancements in our knowledge about aging, children and adults continue making poor lifestyle decisions that accelerate the aging process. People from all age groups and economic levels fail to exercise enough, while eating excessive unhealthy, empty calories. A large percentage of people spend too much time sitting in front of computers, TVs and iPods®, as their muscles atrophy and their weight balloons.

Insufficient vitamins and minerals exacerbate the problem, while negative environmental factors compound these difficulties even more. As we've already shown, toxins from our workplaces, homes, the air, water and food intensify these problematic factors.

Know the risks of a poor diet and toxins

A whopping 95 percent of all cancers result from dietary and environmental toxicities, according to the Columbia University School of Public Health.

Worsening matters, this relentless assault on our body functions leads to multiple chronic illnesses which combine to cause the affects of aging.

As the years pass, people older than 40 experience altered brain function, poor vision and hearing, wrinkling skin and the softening of bones. Other negative impacts include increased body fat and poor posture, plus hardening of the brain, carotid, coronary and peripheral artery system. Besides decreased libido, maturing people suffer difficulties in their livers, kidneys, heart and lung functions.

Even more distressing, the immune system weakens with aging, decreasing the body's ability to fight or ward off potentially debilitating or life-threatening assaults by bacteria, viruses and fungus, or the spread of abnormal cells.

On the positive side, good news emerges as medical professionals and scientists discover that vitamin and mineral supplements and certain foods stop or reverse these negative impacts.

How much vitamins and minerals are recommended?

Most people know that the government recommends a "required daily allowance" or RDA of specific vitamins and minerals. By law, through a required packaging and labeling process, distributors of foods, vitamins and minerals must specify the percentage of these substances that a particular product contains.

However, in all these instances—everything from cereal boxes to milk cartons—the term "100 percent" refers to the *least* amount of a vitamin or mineral that physicians deem necessary to sustain good health. Medical professionals consider these minimum levels as the lowest amounts essential to prevent a wide variety of diseases including scurvy, rickets, pellagra, beriberi, pernicious anemia and many other afflictions.

When developing these FDA requirements, medical professionals used nutritional studies that were conducted as far back as the 1940s. However, at the time scientists and physicians lacked precise methods of testing or determining the levels of vitamins and minerals in tissue and blood. Modern equipment gives much more accurate results.

Sadly, the minimum RDA levels specified by the government fail to meet the human body's requirements, especially amid the increased onslaught of serious cancer, severe cardiovascular disease, environmental toxins and virulent viruses or bacterial illnesses. Severe stress that people under in today's society compounds these problems.

The RDA and optimal daily allowances can vary significantly for specific vitamins or minerals. For instance, the RDA for Vitamin C is 60 milligrams per day, compared to an optimal daily allowance of about 1,000 milligrams daily for the same substance. Vitamins A and E also are among many individual vitamins and minerals with optimal daily doses significantly higher than the RDA listed for each of them.

Make food selection your first level of defense

Considering these many negative factors, the need to adopt a proper food selection or diet program emerges as a primary first step for any serious anti-aging program.

Immediately before starting such a regimen, you should meet a dietary clinician who can determine your ideal weight based on height. In this system known as the body mass index or BMI, the clinician attempts to determine the healthy weight level.

While maintaining a trim, ideal weight might sound merely vane or narcissistic, various medical studies through the years strongly indicate excessive or unnecessary weight contributes to cancer, cardiovascular disease and diabetes mellitus. Maintaining an ideal body weight can go a long way toward preventing or at least lowering the probability of such negative health factors.

The South Beach Diet®, Zone Diet® and Modified Atkin's Diet® already mentioned in the women's health section strive to reduce simple sugars, while increasing proteins and healthy fats. Another food-selection program, the Mediterranean Diet, also has been deemed effective, when consuming meals common from that region.

These diets often prove useful as low-glycemic or in supplying the healthiest form of carbohydrates. Medical professionals can measure the impact that carbohydrates have on blood glucose levels, using a system called the "glycemic index."

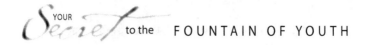

We stress the importance of certain foods

Whenever possible we recommend vegan or near-vegan diets, eliminating or significantly lowering the amount of animals for food. However, occasional broiled or baked lean meats, fowl or fish become acceptable when eaten in lower quantities.

In anti-cancer diets and for weight management, vegetables have proven especially beneficial and healthy, especially cabbage, cauliflower, carrots, beans, broccoli and Brussels sprouts. Foods containing natural digestive enzymes including bromelain from pineapples and papain from papaya are also highly desirable.

All along, you should avoid fried foods, simple sugars, salt, flour and any cured meats such as salami, sausage, bologna, pepperoni, canned meats, Spam®, hot dogs and similar foods. Among other primary foods that we highly recommend to treat or prevent certain aging-related conditions:

- **Citrus foods**: While also helping to prevent cancer, citrus foods containing bioflavonoids, terpenes, limonene and citrus pectin aid the cardiovascular system while serving as antioxidants.

- **Red grapes**: These fruits contain plant flavonoids called "pycnogenol," also present in pine bark extract. Red grapes serve as one of the strongest antioxidants, also helpful in strengthening bone and cartilage tissue while enhancing immune function.

- **Red wine**: This beverage contains resveratrol, which preserves telomere integrity—vital in enabling the body's cells to divide or reproduce with efficiency, thereby promoting longevity.

- **Hawthorne berries**: This food and extracts from such fruits help strengthen bones, tendons, cartilage and cardiac muscle, while serving as a natural treatment for hypertension.

- **Green tea**: Especially in Asia, three or four cups per day have long been known as helpful in preventing cancers—even common killers like lung cancer.

- **Flaxseed lignan fibers**: An excellent hormone regulator, this food source helps protect against breast and prostate cancers.

- **Healthy oils**: Selections such as corn, olive, canola and soy are mono-saturated, important in the production of LDL or good cholesterol.

- **Oat bran and wheat germ**: These natural foods help lower "bad cholesterol," while increasing "good cholesterol."

- **Green "super foods:"** These selections include wheat grass, barley grass and algae, nutrient and trace elements and an excellent source of making the body more alkaline than acidic. These foods also combat acidosis, a hallmark of inflammatory conditions and cancer. (For more on the many benefits of "super food," see the following section on BõKU™ Super Food.)

- **Soybeans**: We know that this excellent anti-aging food, high in protein remains a delight to people who prefer to avoid eating meat. The chemicals in soy contain strong antioxidants, hormone regulators and cancer-prevention qualities, especially in battling breast and prostate cancers. Many people eat soy products, thanks to the cancer-therapeutic properties of these foods.

- **Healthy chocolates**: Derived from natural cocoa, chocolate without sugar or milk products serves as an essential antioxidant. We strongly recommend Xocai™, available via ***ProfitChocolates.com***.

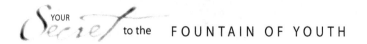

Remember the foods you should eat

While all these various health food opportunities might seem limitless, in summary your food selection list should include: raw or lightly cooked whole grain cereals; raw or lightly steamed vegetables and sprouts; except for citrus selection, raw or fresh fruits including the skin; lightly cooked beans, lentils and peas; preferably unsalted raw nuts and seeds; low-fat dairy products, especially low-fat cultured yogurt; occasional lean meat, fish or poultry, usually limited to one or two times weekly; and an occasional glass of red wine.

Remember the foods you should avoid

The list of foods to avoid remains even more extensive: more than two ounce of alcohol daily, especially whiskey, scotch, vodka and gin; bacon and cured meats; canned or frozen fruits; canned soups; fried foods in any form; all types of gravies; whole milk ice cream; salted peanuts; processed cheese products; processed luncheon meats; saturated fats; soft cheeses; soft drinks and sodas; tuna that is canned in oil; canned or frozen vegetables with salt additives; white or brown sugar; white flour products; white rice products; white vinegar; and fruit syrups.

Avoid high-fat foods

Always remember to avoid foods high in fat content. These include: cake; cookies; doughnuts; ricotta cheese; cream cheese; crescents; regular crackers; breaded or fried fish; whole milk ice cream; butter, mayonnaise; sour cream; de-boned or chuck steaks; dark meat from turkey or chicken; bologna; salami; hot dogs; and sausage.

Take recommended minerals

When following all the various recommendations already mentioned for an anti-aging diet, your body still may need vitamins and minerals from other sources. As a result, you should take the following minerals listed alphabetically:

- **Boron**: This trace mineral activates Vitamin D while aiding the body's ability to absorb and use calcium essential for bone strength and estrogen for the metabolism. Take at lease 3 milligrams daily.

- **Calcium**: As the body's most abundant mineral, this essential substance gets absorbed best in its ionized form such as: citrate: lactate primarily from milk products; gluconate from fruits, honeys, teas and wines; asparatate from sprouting seeds, oat flakes, avocadoes; and orotate. Dietary supplements are often excellent or single sources of calcium. Women, especially shortly before, during and after menopause, should take 1,500 milligrams of calcium daily, usually in three doses of 500 milligrams each.

- **Chromium**: Prevalent in mushrooms, yeast, prunes, nuts and asparagus, this mineral helps sugar metabolism by generating insulin. Without any known toxicity, chromium helps the body lower triglycerides or bad cholesterol. Take at least 400 micrograms daily.

- **Copper**: The body needs this essential trace element for enzyme function or vital biochemical reactions. The body stores or uses most of its copper in the brain or liver. Important in anti-aging therapy, copper's best food sources include fish, dark meat and colored vegetables. Take at least 3 milligrams daily.

- **Magnesium**: This plays an essential role for several hundred enzyme reactions throughout the body. Bones contain 60 percent of the total of this mineral within the body, while muscles have 25 percent. Medical experts find other high concentrations of magnesium in vital organs including the brain, heart, liver and kidneys. Like potassium, most magnesium is intracellular or within the cells. The best magnesium supplements are glycinate, aspartate or taurinate. Common foods that contain magnesium include wheat bran, wheat germ, almonds, cashews, Brazil nuts, peanuts, walnuts, tofu, soybeans and brown rice. Take 400-600 milligrams daily. Excessive quantities may cause diarrhea.

• **Manganese**: Multiple enzyme systems throughout the body use this mineral, necessary for the metabolism's glucose, for energy production, and for thyroid function. Common food sources include nuts, whole grains, split peas, green leafy vegetables and dried fruits. Take 1,500-2,000 milligrams daily.

• **Potassium**: This essential mineral serves vital roles throughout the body, including the performance and functions of the heart and muscles—plus multiple enzyme systems and the balance of electrolyte or free ions within cell structures. Common food sources include bananas, figs, leafy green vegetables and citrus fruits. Take 1,500-2,000 milligrams daily.

• **Selenium**: This essential anti-aging trace mineral serves as a strong antioxidant, acting in concert with Vitamin E to prevent free radicals from damaging cell membranes. Useful in cancer therapy and anti-aging therapy, selenium—proven for its antiviral action—often is recommended for preventing prostate cancer. Physicians also recommend selenium for enhancing immune function and for relieving anxiety. Common food sources include Brazil nuts, sunflower seeds, whole grains, meat products, garlic and seafood. Rare side affects include dizziness, nausea, brittle nails and hair loss. Take 100-200 micrograms daily.

- **Zinc**: Often found in shellfish and red meats, this mineral plays an important role in the functions of vital hormones including insulin, sex hormones, thymus gland hormones, and human growth hormone. Essential for vision, taste and smell, zinc becomes essential for prostate function and male fertility. Especially after surgery, zinc aids protein synthesis and cell growth while also fighting viruses. Citrate, glycerate and picolinate are good zinc supplements. Take 25-50 milligrams daily.

Take anti-aging Vitamin supplements

Antioxidants reign as the most important anti-aging Vitamin supplements, especially Vitamins A, C, E and coenzyme-Q10. Medical professionals consider these vitamins as antioxidants thanks to their unique ability to inactivate free radicals that can accumulate in the body—especially in maturing people.

As explained previously, when left unchecked, free radicals can damage multiple tissues throughout the body, promoting the growth of abnormal cells that can cause cancer or accelerate the signs of aging.

Remember that free radicals become reactive substances formed when energy gets produced. Amid a search for its missing electron, a free radical becomes unstable while randomly attacking healthy molecules in the body. Free radicals cause extensive damage unless stopped by antioxidants.

Worsening matters, free radicals can attack the energy factory or mitochondria, interrupting important enzyme and hormonal systems. This interferes with the body's ability to grow and repair, and to cope with stress.

As a result, antioxidants become necessary to neutralize all free radicals within the body. Among antioxidants that we strongly recommend:

- **Vitamin A and beta-carotene**: Take these together; since beta-carotene causes less toxicity to the liver; you should consider beta-carotene the preferred supplement for Vitamin A. Excellent food sources for beta-carotene include dark leafy vegetables such as spinach, broccoli and peppers—plus dark yellow or orange fruits and vegetables like sweet potatoes, pumpkins, papayas, oranges and apricots. Heavy smokers should avoid large doses of beta-carotene; numerous studies show a propensity for lung cancers among smokers who ingest large doses of beta-carotene and Vitamin A.

- **Vitamin C**: While serving as an excellent antioxidant and anti-aging weapon, Vitamin C strengthens blood vessel walls and promotes wound healing—also stimulating hormonal regulation and brain chemicals. Adding to these many benefits, Vitamin C also increases immune function and protects against toxic chemicals such as potentially cancer-causing nitrosamine chemical compounds. Excellent food sources for Vitamin C include citrus fruits, green or red peppers, broccoli, Brussels sprouts, potatoes, spinach, strawberries, tomatoes and papayas. Rare side affects from Vitamin C include kidney stones. But negative impacts of Vitamin C are rarely seen, even in large doses of 10-15 grams per day; we recommend 1,000-1,500 milligrams daily.

- **Vitamin E:** Along with Vitamin C, this becomes part of a strong anti-aging and antioxidant team. Vitamin E attacks free radicals, blocks the oxygenation of bad cholesterol and other fats, and prevents heart attacks and strokes. Adding to its firepower, Vitamin E keeps arteries free from potentially harmful plaque, increases immunity and blocks the growth of cancer cells. In addition, homeopaths strongly recommend Vitamin E for preventing the progression of degenerative brain diseases, improving the systems related to arthritis, counter-acting

240

cataracts and preventing certain impairments in our ability to walk. Good natural food sources for Vitamin E include seed oils, leafy green vegetables, liver, whole grains, wheat germs, egg yolks, butter and nuts. Vitamin E has a mild ability to prevent blood from clotting. So, you should avoid taking Vitamin E with blood-thinner medications like warfarin and Plavix®. For anti-aging purposes, we recommend 400-800 IU of Vitamin E per day.

- **Coenzyme-Q10**: Also known as Vitamin Q or ubiquinone, this plays an integral role in heart function—particularly congestive heart failure or cardiomyopathy. While lowering blood pressure, Coenzyme-Q10 also enhances the immune system, reduces gum disease and increases energy levels. Common food sources include eggs, rice, bran, wheat germ, fatty fish, organ meats, soy oil and peanuts. Coenzyme-Q10 lacks toxicity side affects. We recommend 300 milligrams daily.

Add the latest supplements to your anti-aging cocktail

Anti-aging medicine becomes fun when we add or mix some or all of these important vitamins with a wide variety of substances that scientists know will slow the signs of aging. Thanks to modern science and cutting-edge production techniques, you can ingest these various substances in supplement form or from certain foods. Listed in alphabetical order, some of the most prevalent include:

- **Acetyl L-Carnitine**: Serves as a powerful antioxidant for the central nervous system and peripheral nerves, in doses of 500 milligrams daily.

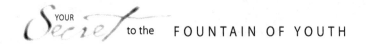

- **Alpha lipoic acid**: An important amino acid essential in transferring energy among cells, this unique antioxidant synergizes, enhances or magnifies B vitamins. Useful in treating various disorders of the central nervous system—called "neuropathies" by physicians—this acid improves the body's regulation of insulin. This, in turn, improves the metabolism and enhances the functions of essential systems like the liver and muscles, recommended at 500 milligrams daily.

- **L-carnitine**: This vitamin-like substance serves a necessary role in helping the body metabolize or process fatty acids, some essential in producing various hormone-like substances. Fatty acids regulate everything from immune responses to blood clotting and even blood pressure. In addition, L-carnitine helps produce energy in the mitochondria, vital in generating the body's essential chemical energy. You should take 4-6 grams daily.

- **Folic acid**: Necessary in the production of neurotransmitters, chemicals that regulate signals between cells and neurons, this substance also enables the body to transfer essential methyl gasses within the body. Working in synergy with Vitamins B6 and B12, folic acid reduces levels of homocysteine—which, in elevated amounts could lead to thrombosis or cardiovascular disease. You should take 400-600 micrograms daily.

- **Ginkgo biloba**: The many positive anti-aging benefits of this extract include improved memory, blood flow to the brain and vascular function. You should use care when using ginkgo biloba, derived from a unique Chinese tree species, and avoid using the extract with blood-thinning agents like warfarin. You should take 60 milligrams daily.

- **L-arginine**: This amino acid stimulates growth hormone production and improves erectile function. You should take 3 grams daily.

- **L-glutamine**: An abundant amino acid, this can work as a "brain fuel" during stressful periods and also serves a vital role in producing muscles and repairing the lining of the intestine. You should take 3 grams daily.

- **L-glutathione**: Hailed by some medical professionals as a "life-extending master antioxidant," this serves a useful role in cancer prevention and in detoxifying the immune system. Also a powerful scavenger of free radicals, L-glutathione serves beneficial roles in treating the conditions of many ailments or physical problems. These include autism, cardiovascular disease, autoimmune diseases, asthma, diabetes, lung disease, colitis, hepatitis, chronic fatigue syndrome, multiple sclerosis, Parkinsonism and Alzheimer's disease. Abundant in the cytoplasm within the plasma membranes of cells and in mitochondria that generate chemical energy, L-glutathione also helps patients with degenerative eye diseases like cataracts and macular degeneration. You should take 100 milligrams daily.

- **Lutein**: Allied with Vitamin A, this substance comes from carotenoids or organic pigments found in various plants. Physicians consider lutein important in preventing and treating prostate cancer and degenerative eye disease. Medical professionals recommend eating natural sources of lutein, including green leafy vegetables, tomatoes, potatoes, spinach, carrots, fruits and algae.

- **Lycopene**: You can find abundant amounts of this powerful antioxidant, anti-cancer substance—also good in treating prostate cancer and degenerative eye diseases—in tomatoes, carrots, green peppers, pink grapefruits and apricots.

- **N-acetylcysteine**: A powerful antioxidant that becomes active when ingested with Vitamin C, medical professionals consider this helpful in brain and cardiac function. You can take 500 milligrams daily.

- **Quercetin**: An antioxidant or bioflavonoid found primarily in plants, this strong anti-viral performs an anti-tumor activity while also helpful to people with severe allergies, asthma and allergic rashes. You can find quercetin in abundance in yellow and red onions and broccoli. You can take 500-1,500 milligrams daily.

- **Turmeric:** Also known as curcumin, abundant in curry powder and mustard, this anti-oxidant with anti-cancer and anti-inflammatory qualities has a positive impact on the intestinal tract plus the immune and cardiovascular systems. You should take 500 milligrams per day.

- **Vitamin B1**: Also called thiamine, working in conjunction with magnesium and found in abundance in coffee and alcohol, this serves a necessary role in optimal brain function. You should take 100 milligrams daily.

- **Vitamin B2**: Commonly called riboflavin, this serves as a natural "glutathione," a term used by physicians to describe something that protects cells from free radicals or toxins. Also vital in the body's energy production, this vitamin is found in abundance in brewers yeast, almonds, wheat germ, mushrooms, whole grains and soy. You should take 30 milligrams daily.

- **Vitamin B3**: Also called niacin, this performs an essential role in 50 enzyme reactions within the body. Besides performing an important role in producing sex hormones and adrenal hormones and energy, niacin performs essential work in metabolizing sugar, fat and cholesterol. You should take 500-1,000 milligrams daily.

- **Vitamin B5**: Also called pantothenic acid, necessary to metabolize sugar and energy, this vitamin plays a necessary role in the production of adrenal hormones and red blood cells. This metabolism process emerges as essential, a process enabling cells to maintain life, grow and reproduce. Working with coenzyme-Q10 and L-carnitine, Vitamin B5 also helps metabolize fat. Excellent food sources include brewers yeast, calf liver, peanuts, mushrooms, soybeans, peas, pecans, oatmeal, sunflower seeds, lentils, oranges and strawberries. You should take 1 gram daily.

- **Vitamin B6**: Commonly called pyridoxine, this plays an important role in regulating neurotransmitters, the chemical process that regulates signals between cells and neurons. Medical professionals also use Vitamin B6 to treat elevated levels of homocysteine, a condition that could—if left unchecked—lead to thrombosis and cardiovascular disease. The body also needs Vitamin B6 for making proteins and for immune system function. Food sources include sunflower seeds, wheat germ, soybeans, walnuts, lentils, beans, whole grains, bananas, spinach, potatoes and cauliflower. You should take 50-100 milligrams daily.

- **Vitamin B12**: Sometimes called cobalamin, this methyl donor responsible in the vital transfer of certain gasses, helps the body maintain cell membranes and neurotransmitters—while also serving a necessary function in the production of normal red blood cells. Vitamin B12 works in synergy with Vitamin B6 and

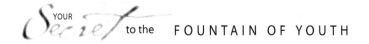

folic acid. You can find Vitamin B12 in abundance in animal foods, liver, lamb meat, shellfish, salmon and cheese. You should take 1,000 micrograms daily.

- **Vitamin D3**: The hydroxyl form of Vitamin D and optimal for cancer prevention, this vitamin displays such power that even allopathic physicians administer doses to breast, prostate and colon cancer patients. You should take 80-100 milligrams daily, or 4,000-6,000 IUs per day.

- **Vitamin K1**: Also called phytonadione and commonly found in green leafy vegetables, this has special anti-aging qualities and aids in treating osteoporosis while important in coagulating blood.

Summary

Exercise, food selections, hormonal supplements, minerals and vitamins play integral roles in the anti-aging process. People who employ a balance of these factors position themselves for healthy, quality-filled aging while lessening the possibility of chronic degenerative diseases like cancer.

APPENDIX 1

James W. Forsythe, M.D., H.M.D.
Board Certified Internal Medicine
Board Certified Medical Oncology
Certified in Homeopathy

This protocol was submitted to the U.S. Food and Drug Administration in 2007 by James W Forsythe, M.D., H.M.D., as part of a settlement agreement with the United States prosecuting attorney's office, Reno, Nevada.

OUTLINE of NATIONAL PROTOCOL

I.   Endorsing organizations
II.   Abbreviations
III.   Mission statement
IV.   Introduction
      a.   Approved products
      b.   Proven Benefits of GHRT
      c.   Cardiovascular risks of GHD
      d.   FDA Aproved Uses of GHRT
      e.   Proposed Expanded Uses of GHRT
V.   Selection of patients
      a.   Appropriate Face-to-Face Work-Up
      b.   Major consideration
VI.   Laboratory testing
      a.   General Facts
      b.   GH Stimulation Tests
      c.   Multiple Endocrine Deficiencies
      d.   IGF-1 and IGF-1-BP-3 Testing
VII.   Therapy Considerations
      a.   FDA Approved Conditions
      b.   Usual Dosages
      c.   Injection Instructions

VIII.   Side-Affects and Adverse Events Profile
        a.   General Facts
        b.   Adult Side-Affects
        c.   Diabetes Facts
IX.   Conclusions
        a.   Obligations to Observe Federal and State Laws
        b.   Expanded Guidelines
        c.   "Off-Label" Pescription
        d.   Overall Benefits of Age-Related GHRT

I.   ENDORSING ORGANIZATIONS
* Academy of Anti-Aging Medicine-China
* Academy of Anti-Aging Medicine-Iberia
* Academy of Healthy Aging
* Academy of Optimal Aging

II.   ABBREVIATIONS
* AACE - American Association of Clinical Endocrinologists
* A4M - American Academy of Anti-Aging Medicine

III.   MISSION STATEMENT

The use of Growth Hormone (GH) in clinical practice is expanding in both clinical endocrinology, as well as the new and expanding discipline of Anti-Aging medicine pioneered mainly by the American Academy of Anti-Aging Medicine (A4M) and the International Hormone Society.

IV.   INTRODUCTION

GH has been used to treat children with GHD for over 40 years.

Endorsing Organizations

- Academy of The Anti-Aging Medicine-China
- Academy of The Anti-Aging Medicine-Iberia
- Academy of Healthy Aging
- Academy of Optimal Aging
- Academy of Successful Aging
- American Academy of Age Management
- American Academy of Anti-Aging Medicine (A4M)
- American Academy of Longevity Medicine
- American College of Longevity Medicine
- American Society of Longevity Medicine
- Anti-Aging Medicine Specialization
- Asian-Oceania Federation of Anti-Aging
- Austral Asian Academy of Anti-Aging Medicine (A5M)
- Belgian Society of Anti-Aging Medicine (BELSAAM)
- European Academy of Quality of Life and Longevity Medicine (EAQUALL)
- European Organization of Scientific Anti-Aging Medicine Anti-Aging
- European Society of Anti-Aging Medicine (ESAAM)
- German Society of Anti-Aging Medicine (GSAAM)
- German Society of Hemotoxicology
- Hellenic Academy of Antiaging Medicine
- Indonesian Society of Anti-Aging Medicine
- International Academy of Anti-Aging Medicine
- International Academy of Longevity Medicine
- International Hormone Society (HIS)
- Japan Anti-Aging Medicine Spa Association (JAMSA)
- Japanese Society of Clinical Anti-Aging Medicine
- Korea Anti-Aging Academy of Medicine (KA3M)
- Latin-American Federation of Anti-Aging Societies
- Romania Association of Anti-Aging Medicine
- Society for Anti-Aging &Aesthetic Medicine Malaysia (SAAAMM)
- South African Academy of Anti-Aging & Aesthetic Medicine (SA5M)
- Spanish Society of Anti-Aging
- Thai Academy of Anti-Aging Medicine

- Thai Association of Anti-Aging Medicine
- Anti-Aging Research and Education Society, Turkey
- Center for Study of Anti-Aging Medicine – UDAYANA University, Indonesia
- World Academy of Anti-Aging Medicine (WAAAM)
- World Academy of Longevity Medicine
- World Society of Anti-Aging Medicine (WOSAAM)

Abbreviations

1. AACE: American Association of Clinical Endocrinologists
2. A4M: American Academy of Anti-Aging Medicine
3. AIDS: Acquired Immunodeficiency syndrome
4. CEA: Carcinoembryonic Antigen
5. DHEA: Dehydroepiandrosterone
6. CFIDS: Chronic Fatigue Immune Dysfunction Syndrome
7. FDA: Federal Food and Drug Administration
8. GH: Growth Hormone
9. GHDS: Growth Hormone Deficiency Syndrome
10. GHRH: Growth Hormone Releasing Hormone
11. GHRT: Growth Hormone Replacement Therapy
12. HGH: Human Growth Hormone
13. HIV: Human Immunodeficiency Virus
14. HRT: Hormone Replacement Therapy(ies)
15. IGFI: Insulin like Growth Factor I
16. IGFBP-3: Insulin like Growth Factor Binding Protein-3
17. MPHD: Multiple Pituitary Hormone Deficiencies
18. PWS: Prader Willi Syndrome
19. SGA: Small for Gestational Age
20. TS: Turner Syndrome

Mission Statement

The use of Growth Hormone (GH) in clinical practice is expanding in both clinical endocrinology and the new and expanding discipline of Anti-Aging medicine pioneered mainly by the American Academy of Anti-Aging Medicine (A4M) and the International Hormone Society. The purpose of this protocol is to establish a national and perhaps an international protocol through the worldwide scientific and medical societies that are dedicated to the appropriate use of GHRT in improving the quality and perhaps the duration of the human lifespan and the function of the individuals physiology and hormonal balance in order to achieve greater vitality, prevention of disease and overall greater health during the aging process.

Admittedly some areas of GHRT will remain controversial until more information and testing becomes available, however, it is the purpose of this protocol to provide the physician with a standard sanctioned by the FDA that allows him to act as an advocate for the patients right for optimal health and freedom of choice in health care.

This protocol consists of recommendations for the clinical use of GHRT. These guidelines should be used by physicians in conjunction with standard history and physical examinations along with appropriate clinical testing in concert with their best clinical judgment.

It is the position of this protocol and its authors that use of GH solely for athletic enhancement constitutes a misuse of this hormone and thereby taints its appropriate usage.

Introduction

GH has been used to treat children with GHD for over 40 years. The original source of HGH was from the pituitary glands of human cadavers. In 1985 it was discovered that this source was subject to contamination with the Creutzfeldt-Jacob virus causing a slowly developing fatal dementia. Fortuitously, about this same time Biosynthetic recombinant GH became available and consequently after 1985 production and distribution of cadaver derived pituitary GH was discontinued.

GH of recombinant DNA origin with an identical 191 amino acid chain sequence is now produced commercially by a number of pharmaceutical companies. At present only the following recombinant HGH products have been approved by the FDA:

PRODUCT	CONDITIONS
Genotropin (Pharmacia)	Pediatric GHD PWS SGA Adult GHD
Humatrope (Lilly)	Pediatric GHD TS Idiopathic short status Adult GHD
Norditropin (Nova Nordisk)	Pediatric GHD Adult GHD
Nutropin (Genentech)	Pediatric GHD TS Adult GHD
Protropin Somatrin (Genentech)	Pediatric GHD
Saizen (Serono)	Pediatric GHD Adult GHD
Serostim (Serono)	AIDS wasting Cachexia
Zorbtive (Serono)	Short Bowel Syndrome
TEV-Tropin (Savient)	Pediatric GHD

The purpose of this protocol is to promote the appropriate application of advanced medical technologies in order to address the changes in hormonal, biochemical, physical and nutritional needs that occurs with the aging process. Over 500 articles in the world's scientific literature supports the benefits claimed by returning hormones to their optimal physiological state when determined by appropriate and reasonable testing to be deficient. It is also a well established scientific premise that many critical hormones either decrease significantly with menopause and andropause but also like GH decline stepwise at a predictable 10-15% per decade after the second decade.

The documented proven benefits of GHRT in adults over the past seventeen years since Daniel Rudman's landmark article in the New England Journal of Medicine in July 1990 includes the following:

1. Increase in lean body mass
2. Loss of body fat mass
3. Improved skin texture and tone
4. Improved lipid profiles (cholesterol, triglycerides, LDL ratio)
5. Improved cardiac ejection fraction
6. Improved bone density
7. Improved exercise tolerance
8. Improved libido
9. Improved sleep quality
10. Improved immune function in patients with HIV

Furthermore the deficiency of GH and IGF-1 leads to an increase in cardiovascular risk factors. These include:

1. Increase in visceral fat
2. Increase in carotid intima/media thickness
3. Increase clotting factors
4. Increase in serum CRP
5. Increase in insulin resistance
6. Increase in serum homocysteine

Adult GHD has been associated with an increased risk of fatal stroke and myocardial infarction.

At the present time the only FDA approved "on label" or "medically necessary" uses of GHRT are for patients with the following conditions:

1. Follow-up treatment for documented GHD in childhood
2. Documented hypopituitarism as a result of pituitary or hypothalamic disease from tumors, surgery, radiation therapy or trauma
3. AIDS Wasting Syndrome
4. Short Bowel Syndrome

It is the objective of this protocol to expand the "on label" and "medically necessary" uses of GHRT to include:

1. Therapy in adults over the age of 40 with normally occurring decreases in GH known as age-related GHD.

2. Treatment of congestive cardiomyopathies and congestive heart failure
3. Treatment of severe burn patients
4. Treatment of patients with severe Chronic Fatigue Immune Dysfunction Syndrome (CFIDS) and / or fibromyalgia (FM)
5. Treatment of morbid obesity
6. Traumatic of Brain Injury (TBI)

Selection of Patients

The same concerns that exist in any other area of medicine apply in the field of GHRT. These include:

1. A history of documented hormonal deficiencies
2. Signs and symptoms consistent with a deficiency state: i.e. easy fatigue. lack of energy, decreased libido, poor exercise tolerance, sleep disturbances, etc...
3. Review of medical records to document prior hormonal replacement therapies
4. History of pituitary tumors, surgery, radiation therapy, trauma or prior chemotherapy

This protocol recommends a complete and comprehensive medical history, review of systems as well as a thorough physical examination.

The major contraindications to GHRT are:

1. Active cancer patients
2. Patients with type I and II Diabetes Mellitus (relative contraindication)
3. Patients with metabolic syndrome (relative contraindication)
4. Patients with carpal tunnel syndrome

Laboratory Testing

In general it is the medical judgment of each physician based on a thorough comprehensive medical history, review of symptoms/systems, physical and laboratory testing to determine the medical necessity of prescribing GHRT. Unfortunately with GHD there is no single perfect and reliable test to measure GHD. GHD has a short half-life of less than 20 minutes in the blood and is produced mainly during deep REM sleep thus making it impracticable to directly test for GH itself. Short of this the next most reliable and practical test is another hormone whose production is predominantly stimulated by growth hormones called IGF-1 (Insulin-like growth

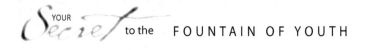

to the FOUNTAIN OF YOUTH

factor 1) and which level is relatively stable in blood throughout the day. Even more reliable is the ratio between IGF-1 and its major binding protein IGF-BP-3 (IGF-1 binding protein 3). This ration provides a better picture of the amount of bioavailable IGF-1 for the target cells. The higher the ratio IGF-1/IGF-BP-3 the more IGF-1 is available for the target cells. A 24 hour hGH urine determination.

1. Arginine
2. GHRH (Growth Hormone Releasing Hormone)
3. Clonidine
4. Glucagon
5. L-Dopa
6. Insulin
7. Propanolol

All of these are cumbersome and puts some patients at unnecessary and unacceptable risks for little diagnostic return. The Insulin Tolerance Test is felt to be the best predictor of GHD. Failure to respond to insulin-induced hypoglycemia is indicative of GHD but carries all the risks of hypoglycemia-i.e. sweats, nausea, vomiting, mental aberrations, hypotension and possible seizures. Of note, if the patient has coronary artery disease the insulin stimulation test is contraindicated.

Along with a low serum IGF-1 level the documented presence of at least three other pituitary deficiencies (i.e. ACTH, TSH, LH) is, in itself, an indication for GHRT.

In summary the IGF-1 level, especially if documented to be below 200 on two separate testing days, is the most practical cost effective and safest test. The International Hormone Society, the world's third largest physician endocrine society, (www.intlhormonesociety.org) and the A4M (www.worldhealth.net) recommends levels in the 300 – 350 microgram/liter range for serum IGF-1 as optimal for average sized men, while a slightly lower level of 250 – 300 is recommended for a median sized woman. Taller or bigger persons may need a higher level, while smaller and thinner persons a lower serum IGF-1 level. The best IGF-1–BP-3 is an average level, around the 3,000 microgram/ liter mark.

Regardless of which stimulation test is used the cutoff point of 5 micrograms/liter is used for all provocative stimulation tests.

The clinician should be aware that IGF-1 levels may be reduced by poor nutrition, hepatic disease, severe diabetes mellitus, sex hormone deficiencies and untreated hypothyroidism.

Measurements of IGF binding protein (IGFBP-3) alone have thus far not been proven to offer superior results than IGF-1 testing alone.

Therapy Considerations

In 1996 the FDA approved GH for use in adult patients with GHD. In addition to the aforementioned indications there is a small group of patients with other kinds of pituitary-hypothalamic diseases including Sheehan's Syndrome, auto-immune hypophysitis and sarcoidosis.

Initiation and titration of GHRT is left to the skill and care of the individual doctor trained in GHRT. Recombinant HGH is dispensed in mgm doses where 1.0mg equals 3 units. The usual starting dose is 0.1mgm to 0.3mgm subcutaneously per day.
Injections are best given at night 5-7 days per week using a ¼ inch number 25 or 27 gauge needle perpendicular to midwaist pinched fatty tissue.

Side Effects and Adverse Events Profile

In general, the risks of GHRT are exceedingly low especially in studies where a low dose fixed regimen is used at bedtime or in divided daily doses.

In the clinical setting as promoted by The International Hormone Society and the A4M, adult GHRT employs doses that are 1/7th (one seventh) the pediatric dose schedule. For a 70 kg man the usual dose would be 0.05 mg to 0.56 mg per day.

When side effects do occur they disappear with cessation of treatment. These include arthralgias, female breast fullness, mild hand numbness (carpal tunnel like symptoms), mild fluid retention and transient elevation of blood sugar levels.

While adult GHRT may cause transient blood sugar elevation during the course of the first months of treatment this does not go on to irreversible diabetes mellitus. In small long-term GH treatment studies a decrease in glycosylated hemoglobin, a marker of diabetes has been reported thanks to the increase in lean body mass and the decrease of body fat mass provided by GHRT. There is no study showing GHRT leads to a permanent diabetic state.

Promotion of cancer by GHRT has long been a concern of endocrinologists and The International Hormone Society and the A4M, however the following data refute this hypothesis:

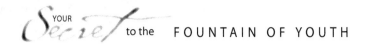

1. Acromegaly patients do not have higher cancer rates than the general population
2. Pediatric GHD patients on long-term GHHRT have not shown an increased cancer incidence
3. As GH declines with age the rate of cancer increases
4. By stimulating improved immune function cancer rates should be reduced

In summary, GHRT is associated with negligible side effects when administered judiciously by a qualified physician.

Conclusions

The authors of this protocol do not endorse or condone the prescription or dispensation of controlled substances or any prescription drugs outside the scope of a bona fide physician-patient relationship. It is incumbent upon every practitioner to comply with the obligations imposed by federal and state laws and regulations in this area.

This protocol has presented the general guidelines and proposed expanded uses of GH for age related adult GHD syndrome. A 70 year old patient may have an IGF-1 level 20% that of a 20-30 year old patient. Physicians replace all other hormonal deficiencies (thyroid, sex hormones, adrenal hormones, etc.) with impunity and without the threat of criminal indictments but GH because it was wrongly included in the Anabolic Steroids Control Act of 1990 and not the Controlled Substance Act became a forbidden treatment for the natural and predictable stepwise decrease in quantity during the aging process. In March 2007, a bill was introduced into the U.S. Senate to amend the Controlled Substance Act (CSA) and to add HGH to schedule III. If we use the argument that hormonal decline is a natural part of aging then as doctors we must explain why we replace sex hormones during menopause and andropause and thyroid hormones in mid life.

The FDA has recognized that "off-label" prescribing is a legitimate part of the practice of medicine and that the practice of medicine is regulated by the State Boards and not by the FDA. The pharmaceutical industry has recently reported that 50% of all general prescriptions are "off-label" and in Oncology it is 80%. It is the physicians ethical responsible to provide the best care for their patients.

This protocol is proposing an "on label" usage of HGH in age related GHD to serve as a prevention for heart disease, cardiovascular disease, osteoarthritis, obesity and in general a healthier aging population. A more widespread usage of age related GHD replacement therapy would also reduce health care costs and give patients the opportunity for higher quality of life during the aging process.

This protocol is submitted by James W Forsythe, MD, HMD as part of a settlement agreement with the United States prosecuting attorney's office, Reno, Nevada.

References

I) <u>MILDER FORMS OF GROWTH HORMONE DEFICIENCY gradually appear with age in adults</u>

because of the gradual aging and thus age-related decline of the pituitary gland.

Senescence is associated with lower GH and IGF-1 levels and increased somatostatin

1. Rudman D, Kutner MH, Rogers CM, Lubin MF, Fleming GA, Bain RP. Impaired growth hormone secretion in the adult population: relation to age and adiposity. J Clin Invest. 1981 May;67(5):1361-9
2. Bando H, Zhang C, Takada Y, Yamasaki R, Saito S. Impaired secretion of growth hormone-releasing hormone, growth hormone and IGF-I in elderly men. Acta Endocrinol (Copenh). 1991 Jan;124(1):31-3
3. Iranmanesh A, Lizarralde G, Veldhuis JD. Age and relative adiposity are specific negative determinants of the frequency and amplitude of growth hormone (GH) secretory bursts and the half-life of endogenous GH in healthy men. J Clin Endocrinol Metab. 1991 Nov;73(5):1081-8
4. Rudman D, Rao UMP. The hypothalamic–growth hormone–somatomedin C axis: The effect of Aging. In: Endocrinology & Metabolism in the Elderly 1992, Eds Morley JC & Korenman SO, Blackwell Sc Publ, Boston-USA
5. Rolandi E, Franceschini R, Marabini A, Messina V, Cataldi A, Salvemini M, Barreca T. Twenty-four-hour beta-endorphin secretory pattern in the elderly. Acta Endocrinol (Copenh). 1987 Aug;115(4):441-6

Senescence is associated with alterations in the circadian cycle of serum GH:

a reduced amplitude and aphase advance
6. Mazzoccoli G, Correra M, Bianco G, De Cata A, Balzanelli M, Giuliani A, Tarquini R. Age-related changes of neuro-endocrine-immune interactions in healthy humans. J Biol Regul Homeost Agents. 1997 Oct-Dec;11(4):143-7

II) SUPPORTING DATA ON GROWTH HORMONE'S BENEFICIAL EFFECTS IN ADULTS

1) GH is important for psychic well-being

Lower quality of life and fatigue: the association with lower GH and/or IGF-1 levels

7.   Gilchrist FJ, Murray RD, Shalet SM. The effect of long-term untreated growth hormone deficiency (GHD) and 9 years of GH replacement on the quality of life (QoL) of GH-deficient adults. Clin Endocrinol (Oxf). 2002 Sep;57(3):363-70

8.   Abs R, Bengtsson BA, Hernberg-Stahl E, Monson JP, Tauber JP, Wilton P, Wuster C. GH replacement in 1034 growth hormone deficient hypopituitary adults: demographic and clinical characteristics, dosing and safety. Clin Endocrinol (Oxf). 1999 Jun;50(6):703-13

9.   Murray RD, Skillicorn CJ, Howell SJ, Lissett CA, Rahim A, Shalet SM. Dose titration and patient selection increases the efficacy of GH replacement in severely GH deficient adults. Clin Endocrinol (Oxf). 1999 Jun;50(6):749-57

Lower quality of life and fatigue: the effect of GH and/or IGF-1 treatment

10.   Murray RD, Darzy KH, Gleeson HK, Shalet SM. GH-deficient survivors of childhood cancer: GH replacement during adult life. J Clin Endocrinol Metab. 2002 Jan;87(1):129-35

11.   Murray RD, Skillicorn CJ, Howell SJ, Lissett CA, Rahim A, Smethurst LE, Shalet SM. Influences on quality of life in GH deficient adults and their effect on response to treatment. Clin Endocrinol (Oxf). 1999 Nov;51(5):565-73

12.   Ahmad AM, Hopkins MT, Thomas J, Ibrahim H, Fraser WD, Vora JP. Body composition and quality of life in adults with growth hormone deficiency; effects of low-dose growth hormone replacement. Clin Endocrinol (Oxf). 2001 Jun;54(6):709-17

13.   Davies JS, Obuobie K, Smith J, Rees DA, Furlong A, Davies N, Evans LM, Scanlon MF. A therapeutic trial of growth hormone in hypopituitary adults and its influence upon continued prescription by general practitioners. Clin Endocrinol (Oxf) 2000 Mar;52(3):295-303

14.   McGauley GA Quality of life assessment before and after growth hormone treatment in adults with growth hormone deficiency. Acta Paediatr Scand Suppl. 1989;356:70-2

15.   Cuneo RC, Judd S, Wallace JD, Perry-Keene D, Burger H, Lim-Tio S, Strauss B, Stockigt J, Topliss D, Alford F, Hew L, Bode H, Conway A, Handelsman

D, Dunn S, Boyages S, Cheung NW, Hurley D. The Australian Multicenter Trial of Growth Hormone (GH) Treatment in GH-Deficient Adults. J Clin Endocrinol Metab. 1998 Jan;83(1):107-16

16. Li Voon Chong JS, Benbow S, Foy P, Wallymahmed ME, Wile D, MacFarlane IA. Elderly people with hypothalamic-pituitary disease and growth hormone deficiency: lipid profiles, body composition and quality of life compared with control subjects. Clin Endocrinol (Oxf). 2000 Nov;53(5):551-9

17. Moorkens G, Berwaerts J, Wynants H, Abs R. Characterization of pituitary function with emphasis on GH secretion in the chronic fatigue syndrome. Clin Endocrinol (Oxf). 2000 Jul;53(1):99-106

18. Wallymahmed ME, Baker GA, Humphris G, Dewey M, MacFarlane IA. The development, reliability and validity of a disease specific quality of life model for adults with growth hormone deficiency. Clin Endocrinol (Oxf). 1996 Apr;44(4):403-11

19. Lagrou K, Xhrouet-Heinrichs D, Massa G, Vandeweghe M, Bourguignon JP, De Schepper J, de Zegher F, Ernould C, Heinrichs C, Malvaux P, Craen M. Quality of life and retrospective perception of the effect of growth hormone treatment in adult patients with childhood growth hormone deficiency. J Pediatr Endocrinol Metab. 2001;14 Suppl 5:1249-60

20. Stabler B. Impact of growth hormone (GH) therapy on quality of life along the lifespan of GH-treated patients. Horm Res. 2001;56 Suppl 1:55-8

21. Wiren L, Johannsson G, Bengtsson BA. A prospective investigation of quality of life and psychological well-being after the discontinuation of GH treatment in adolescent patients who had GH deficiency during childhood. J Clin Endocrinol Metab. 2001 Aug;86(8):3494-8

22. Bjork S, Jonsson B, Westphal O, Levin JE. Quality of life of adults with growth hormone deficiency: a controlled study. Acta Paediatr Scand Suppl 1989;356:55-9; discussion 60, 73-4

23. Bengtsson BA, Abs R, Bennmarker H, Monson JP, Feldt-Rasmussen U, Hernberg-Stahl E, Westberg B, Wilton P, Wuster C. The effects of treatment and the individual responsiveness to growth hormone (GH) replacement therapy in 665 GH-deficient adults. KIMS Study Group and the KIMS International Board. J Clin Endocrinol Metab 1999 Nov;84(11):3929-35

24. Laron Z. Consequences of not treating children with Laron syndrome (primary growth hormone insensitivity). J Pediatr Endocrinol Metab. 2001;14 Suppl 5:1243-8; discussion 1261-2

25. Page RC, Hammersley MS, Burke CW, Wass JA. An account of the quality of life of patients after treatment for non-functioning pituitary tumours. Clin Endocrinol (Oxf). 1997 Apr;46(4):401-6

Lower quality of life and fatigue: the improvement with GH treatment

26. Wallymahmed ME, Foy P, Shaw D, Hutcheon R, Edwards RH, MacFarlane IA. Quality of life, body composition and muscle strength in adult growth hormone deficiency: the influence of growth hormone replacement therapy for up to 3 years. Clin Endocrinol (Oxf). 1997 Oct;47(4):439-46

27. Kozakowski J, Adamkiewicz M, Krassowski J, Zgliczynski S. The beneficial effects of growth hormone replacement therapy on elderly men. Pol Merkuriusz Lek. 1999 Mar;6(33):131-4

28. Waters D, Danska J, Hardy K, Koster F, Qualls C, Nickell D, Nightingale S, Gesundheit N, Watson D, Schade D. Recombinant human growth hormone, insulin-like growth factor 1, and combination therapy in AIDS-associated wasting. A randomized, double-blind, placebo-controlled trial. Ann Intern Med. 1996 Dec 1;125(11):865-72

29. Bengtsson BA, Abs R, Bennmarker H, Monson JP, Feldt-Rasmussen U, Hernberg-Stahl E, Westberg B, Wilton P, Wuster C. The effects of treatment and the individual responsiveness to growth hormone (GH) replacement therapy in 665 GH-deficient adults. KIMS Study Group and the KIMS International Board. J Clin Endocrinol Metab. 1999 Nov;84(11):3929-35

30. Feldt-Rasmussen U, Abs R, Bengtsson BA, Bennmarker H, Bramnert M, Hernberg-Stahl E, Monson JP, Westberg B, Wilton P, Wuster C; KIMS International Study Board on behalf of KIMS Study Group.Growth hormone deficiency and replacement in hypopituitary patients previously treated for acromegaly or Cushing's disease. Eur J Endocrinol. 2002 Jan;146(1):67-74

31. Hernberg-Stahl E, Luger A, Abs R, Bengtsson BA, Feldt-Rasmussen U, Wilton P, Westberg B, Monson JP; KIMS International Board.; KIMS Study Group. Pharmacia International Metabolic Database. Healthcare consumption decreases in parallel with improvements in quality of life during GH replacement in hypopituitary adults with GH deficiency. J Clin Endocrinol Metab. 2001 Nov;86(11):5277-81

32. Wiren L, Bengtsson BA, Johannsson G. Beneficial effects of long-term GH replacement therapy on quality of life in adults with GH deficiency. Clin Endocrinol (Oxf). 1998 May;48(5):613-20

33. Fazio S, Sabatini D, Capaldo B, Vigorito C, Giordano A, Guida R, Pardo F, Biondi B, Sacca L.A preliminary study of growth hormone in the treatment of dilated cardiomyopathy. N Engl J Med. 1996 Mar 28;334(13):809-14

34. Burman P, Deijen JB. Quality of life and cognitive function in patients with pituitary insufficiency. Psychother Psychosom. 1998;67(3):154-67

35. Carroll PV, Littlewood R, Weissberger AJ, Bogalho P, McGauley G, Sonksen PH, Russell-Jones DL. The effects of two doses of replacement growth hormone on the biochemical, body composition and psychological profiles of growth hormone-deficient adults. Eur J Endocrinol. 1997 Aug;137(2):146-53

36.   54. Burman P, Broman JE, Hetta J, Wiklund I, Erfurth EM, Hagg E, Karlsson FA. Quality of life in adults with growth hormone (GH) deficiency: response to treatment with recombinant human GH in a placebo-controlled 21-month trial. J Clin Endocrinol Metab. 1995 Dec;80(12):3585-90

Depression: the association with lower GH and/or IGF-1 levels

37.   Jarrett DB, Miewald JM, Kupfer DJ. Recurrent depression is associated with a persistent reduction in sleep-related growth hormone secretion. Arch Gen Psychiatry. 1990 Feb;47(2):113-8
38.   Jarrett DB, Kupfer DJ, Miewald JM, Grochocinski VJ, Franz B. Sleep-related growth hormone secretion is persistently suppressed in women with recurrent depression: a preliminary longitudinal analysis. J Psychiatr Res. 1994 May-Jun;28(3):211-23)
39.   Rubin RT, Poland RE, Lesser IM. Neuroendocrine aspects of primary endogenous depression. X: Serum growth hormone measures in patients and matched control subjects. Biol Psychiatry. 1990 May 15;27(10):1065-82
40.   Schilkrut R, Chandra O, Osswald M, Ruther E, Baafusser B, Matussek. Growth hormone release during sleep and with thermal stimulation in depressed patients. Neuropsychobiology. 1975;1(2):70-9
41.   Barry S, Dinan TG. Neuroendocrine challenge tests in depression: a study of growth hormone, TRH and cortisol release. J Affect Disord. 1990 Apr;18(4):229-34
42.   Dinan TG, Barry S. Responses of growth hormone to desipramine in endogenous and non-endogenous depression. Br J Psychiatry. 1990 May;156:680-4
43.   Voderholzer U, Laakmann G, Wittmann R, Daffner-Bujia C, Hinz A, Haag C, Baghai T. Profiles of spontaneous 24-hour and stimulated growth hormone secretion in male patients with endogenous depression. Psychiatry Res. 1993 Jun;47(3):215-27
44.   Harro J, Rimm H, Harro M, Grauberg M, Karelson K, Viru AM. Association of depressiveness with blunted growth hormone response to maximal physical exercise in young healthy men. Psychoneuroendocrinology. 1999 Jul;24(5):505-17
45.   Greden JF. Biological markers of melancholia and reclassification of depressive disorders. Encephale. 1982;8(2):193-202
46.   McMillan CV, Bradley C, Gibney J, Healy ML, Russell-Jones DL, Sonksen PH. Psychological effects of withdrawal of growth hormone therapy from adults with growth hormone deficiency. Clin Endocrinol. (Oxf). 2003 Oct;59(4):467-75

Depression: the improvement with GH treatment

47. Mahajan T, Crown A, Checkley S, Farmer A, Lightman S. Atypical depression in growth hormone deficient adults, and the beneficial effects of growth hormone treatment on depression and quality of life. Eur J Endocrinol. 2004 Sep;151(3):325-32

48. Johansson JO, Larson G, Andersson M, Elmgren A, Hynsjo L, Lindahl A, Lundberg PA, Isaksson OG, Lindstedt S, Bengtsson BA. Treatment of growth hormone-deficient adults with recombinant human growth hormone increases the concentration of growth hormone in the cerebrospinal fluid and affects neurotransmitters. Neuroendocrinology. 1995 Jan;61(1):57-66 *(GH increases endorphins, reduces dopamine)*

Anxiety: the association with lower GH and/or IGF-1 levels

49. Tancer ME, Stein MB, Uhde TW. Growth hormone response to intravenous clonidine in social phobia: comparison to patients with panic disorder and healthy volunteers. Biol Psychiatry. 1993 Nov 1;34(9):591-5

50. Cameron OG, Abelson JL, Young EA. Anxious and depressive disorders and their comorbidity: effect on central nervous system noradrenergic function. Biol Psychiatry. 2004 Dec 1;56(11):875-83

51. Stabler B. Impact of growth hormone (GH) therapy on quality of life along the lifespan of GH-treated patients. Horm Res. 2001;56 Suppl 1:55-8

52. Abelson JL, Glitz D, Cameron OG, Lee MA, Bronzo M, Curtis GC. Blunted growth hormone response to clonidine in patients with generalized anxiety disorder. Arch Gen Psychiatry. 1991 Feb;48(2):157-62

Anxiety: the improvement with GH treatment

53. Arwert LI, Deijen JB, Muller M, Drent ML. Long-term growth hormone treatment preserves GH-induced memory and mood improvements: a 10-year follow-up study in GH-deficient adult men. Horm Behav. 2005 Mar;47(3):343-9

54. Lasaite L, Bunevicius R, Lasiene D, Lasas L. Psychological functioning after growth hormone therapy in adult growth hormone deficient patients: endocrine and body composition correlates. Medicina (Kaunas). 2004;40(8):740-4

Memory loss and Alzheimer's disease: the association with lower GH and/or IGF-1 levels

55. Deijen JB, de Boer H, Blok GJ, van der Veen EA. Cognitive impairments and mood disturbances in growth hormone deficient men.

Psychoneuroendocrinology. 1996 Apr;21(3):313-22
56. Rollero A, Murialdo G, Fonzi S, Garrone S, Gianelli MV, Gazzerro E, Barreca A, Polleri A. Relaionship between cognitive function, growth hormone and insulin-like growth factor I plasma levels in aged subjects. Neuropsychobiology. 1998;38(2):73-9
57. van Dam PS, de Winter CF, de Vries R, van der Grond J, Drent ML, Lijffijt M, Kenemans JL, Aleman A, de Haan EH, Koppeschaar HP. Childhood-onset growth hormone deficiency, cognitive function and brain N-acetylaspartate. Psychoneuroendocrinology. 2005 May;30(4):357-63
58. Watanabe T, Koba S, Kawamura M, Itokawa M, Idei T, Nakagawa Y, Iguchi T, Katagiri T. Small dense low-density lipoprotein and carotid atherosclerosis in relation to vascular dementia. Metabolism. 2004 Apr;53(4):476-82

Memory loss and Alzheimer's disease: the improvement with GH treatment

59. Deijen JB, de Boer H, van der Veen EA. Cognitive changes during growth hormone replacement in adult men. Psychoneuroendocrinology. 1998 Jan;23(1):45-55
60. Koppeschaar HP. Growth hormone, insulin-like growth factor I and cognitive function in adults. Growth Horm IGF Res. 2000 Apr;10 Suppl B:S69-73

Sleep disorders: the association with lower GH and/or IGF-1 levels

61. Astrom C, Lindholm J. Growth hormone-deficient young adults have decreased deep sleep. Neuroendocrinology. 1990 Jan;51(1):82-4

Sleep disorders: the improvement with GH treatment

62. Astrom C, Pedersen SA, Lindholm J. The influence of growth hormone on sleep in adults with growth hormone deficiency. Clin Endocrinol (Oxf). 1990 Oct;33(4):495-500

Loss of sexual drive, sensitivity and/or potency: the association with lower GH and/or IGF-1 levels

63. Becker AJ, Uckert S, Stief CG, Scheller F, Knapp WH, Hartmann U, Brabant G, Jonas U. Serum levels of human growth hormone during different penile conditions in the cavernous and systemic blood of healthy men and patients with erectile dysfunction. Urology. 2002 Apr;59(4):609-14
64. Huang X, Li S, Hu L. Growth hormone deficiency and age-related erectile dysfunction. Zhonghua Nan Ke Xue. 2004 Nov;10(11):867

Loss of sexual potency: the improvement with GH treatment

65.   Becker AJ, Uckert S, Stief CG, Truss MC, Machtens S, Scheller F, Knapp WH, Hartmann U, Jonas U. Possible role of human growth hormone in penile erection. J Urol. 2000 Dec;164(6):2138-42
66.   Zhang XS, Wang YX, Han YF, Li Z, Xiang ZQ, Leng J, Huang XY. Effects of growth hormone supplementation on erectile function and expression of nNOS in aging rats. Zhonghua Nan Ke Xue. 2005 May;11(5):339-42
67.   Jung GW, Spencer EM, Lue TF. Growth hormone enhances regeneration of nitric oxide synthase-containing penile nerves after cavernous nerve neurotomy in rats. J Urol. 1998 Nov;160(5):1899-904

2) GH is important for the good physical appearance and body composition

Sarcopenia: the association with lower GH and/or IGF-1 levels

68.   Sartorio A, Narici MV. Growth hormone (GH) treatment in GH-deficient adults: effects on muscle size,strength and neural activation. Clin Physiol 1994 Sep;14(5):527-37
69.   De Boer H, Blok GJ, Voerman HJ, De Vries PM, van der Veen EA. Body composition in adult growth hormone-deficient men, assessed by anthropometry and bioimpedance analysis. J Clin Endocrinol Metab 1992 Sep;75(3):833-7
70.   Cuneo RC, Salomon F, Wiles CM, Hesp R, Sonksen PH. Growth hormone treatment in growth hormone-deficient adults. I. Effects on muscle mass and strength. J Appl Physiol 1991 Feb;70(2):688-94

Sarcopenia: the improvement with GH treatment

71.   Vahl N, Juul A, Jorgensen JO, Orskov H, Skakkebaek NE, Christiansen JS. Continuation of growth hormone (GH) replacement in GH-deficient patients during transition from childhood to adulthood: a two-year placebo-controlled study. J Clin Endocrinol Metab. 2000 May;85(5):1874-81
72.   Butterfield GE, Marcus R, Holloway L, Butterfield G. Clinical use of growth hormone in elderly people. J Reprod Fertil Suppl. 1993; 46:115-8
73.   Butterfield GE, Thompson J, Rennie MJ, Marcus R, Hintz RL, Hoffman AR. Effect of rhGH and rhIGF-1 treatment on protein utilization in elderly women. Am J Physiol. 1997 Jan; 272 (1 Pt 1): E 94-9
74.   Sartorio A, Narici MV. Growth hormone (GH) treatment in GH-deficient adults: effects on muscle size,strength and neural activation. Clin Physiol. 1994 Sep;14(5):527-37

75. Janssen YJ, Doornbos J, Roelfsema F. Changes in muscle volume, strength, and bioenergetics during recombinant human ,growth hormone (GH) therapy in adults with GH deficiency. J Clin Endocrinol Metab. 1999 Jan;84(1):279-84

76. Jorgensen JO, Pedersen SA, Thuesen L, Jorgensen J, Ingemann-Hansen T, Skakkebaek NE, Christiansen JS. Beneficial effects of growth hormone treatment in GH-deficient adults. Lancet. 1989 Jun 3;1(8649):1221-5

77. ter Maaten JC, de Boer H, Kamp O, Stuurman L, van der Veen EA. Long-term effects of growth hormone (GH) replacement in men with childhood-onset GH deficiency. J Clin Endocrinol Metab. 1999 Jul;84(7):2373-80

78. Whitehead HM, Boreham C, McIlrath EM, Sheridan B, Kennedy L, Atkinson AB, Hadden DR. Growth hormone treatment of adults with growth hormone deficiency: results of a 13-month placebo controlled cross-over study. Clin Endocrinol (Oxf). 1992 Jan;36(1):45-52

79. Nam SY, Kim KR, Cha BS, Song YD, Lim SK, Lee HC, Huh KB. Low-dose growth hormone treatment combined with diet restriction decreases insulin resistance by reducing visceral fat and increasing muscle mass in obese type 2 diabetic patients. Int J Obes Relat Metab Disord. 2001 Aug;25(8):1101-7

Lean body mass: the association with lower GH and/or IGF-1 levels

80. De Boer H, Blok GJ, Voerman HJ, De Vries PM, van der Veen EA. Body composition in adult growth hormone-deficient men, assessed by anthropometry and bioimpedance analysis. J Clin Endocrinol Metab. 1992 Sep;75(3):833-7

Lean body mass: the improvement with GH treatment

81. Bengtsson BA, Eden S, Lonn L, Kvist H, Stokland A, Lindstedt G, Bosaeus I, Tolli J, Sjostrom L, Isaksson OG. Treatment of adults with growth hormone (GH) deficiency with recombinant human GH. J Clin Endocrinol Metab. 1993 Feb;76(2):309-17

82. Lombardi G, Luger A, Marek J, Russell-Jones D, Sonksen P, Attanasio AF. Short-term safety and efficacy of human GH replacement therapy in 595 adults with GH deficiency: a comparison of two dosage algorithms. J Clin Endocrinol Metab. 2002 May;87(5):1974-9

83. Vahl N, Juul A, Jorgensen JO, Orskov H, Skakkebaek NE, Christiansen JS. Continuation of growth hormone (GH) replacement in GH-deficient patients during transition from childhood to adulthood: a two-year placebo-controlled study. J Clin Endocrinol Metab. 2000 May;85(5):1874-81

84. Rudman D, Feller AG, Nagraj HS, Gergans GA, Lalitha PY, Goldberg AF, Schlenker RA, Cohn L, Rudman IW, Mattson DE. Effects of human growth

hormone in men over 60 years old. N Engl J Med. 1990 Jul 5;323(1):1-6

85. Davies JS, Obuobie K, Smith J, Rees DA, Furlong A, Davies N, Evans LM, Scanlon MF. A therapeutic trial of growth hormone in hypopituitary adults and its influence upon continued prescription by general practitioners. Clin Endocrinol (Oxf). 2000 Mar;52(3):295-303

86. Olsovska V, Siprova H, Beranek M, Soska V. The influence of long-term growth hormone replacement therapy on body composition, bone tissue and some metabolic parameters in adults with growth hormone deficiency. Vnitr Lek. 2005 Dec;51(12):1356-*64*

Physical appearance, body morphology improvement with GH treatment

87. Hertoghe T. Growth hormone therapy in aging adults. Anti-aging Med Ther. 1997;1:10-28

88. Zivicnjak M, Franke D, Ehrich JH, Filler G.Does growth hormone therapy harmonize distorted morphology and body composition in chronic renal failure? Pediatr Nephrol. 2000 Dec;15(3-4):229-35

89. Eiholzer U, Schlumpf M, Nordmann Y, l'Allemand D. Early manifestations of Prader-Willi syndrome: influence of growth hormone. J Pediatr Endocrinol Metab 2001;14 Suppl 6:1441-4

3) GH may protect – at least partially - against the appearance of age-related diseases

Hypercholesterolemia: the association with lower GH and/or IGF-1 levels

90. Abdu TA, Neary R, Elhadd TA, Akber M, Clayton RN. Coronary risk in growth hormone deficient hypopituitary adults: increased predicted risk is due largely to lipid profile abnormalities. Clin Endocrinol (Oxf) 2001 Aug;55(2):209-16

91. Landin-Wilhelmsen K, Wilhelmsen L, Lappas G, Rosen T, Lindstedt G, Lundberg PA, Bengtsson BA. Serum insulin-like growth factor I in a random population sample of men and women: relation to age, sex, smoking habits, coffee consumption and physical activity, blood pressure and concentrations of plasma lipids, fibrinogen, parathyroid hormone and osteocalcin. Clin Endocrinol (Oxf). 1994 Sep;41(3):351-7

92. Sanmarti A, Lucas A, Hawkins F, Webb SM, Ulied A. Observational study in adult hypopituitary patients with untreated growth hormone deficiency (ODA study). Socio-economic impact and health status. Collaborative ODA (Observational GH Deficiency in Adults) Group. Eur J Endocrinol. 1999 Nov;141(5):481-9

93. Colao A, di Somma C, Pivonello R, Cuocolo A, Spinelli L, Bonaduce D,

Salvatore M, Lombardi G. The cardiovascular risk of adult GH deficiency (GHD) improved after GH replacement and worsened in untreated GHD: a 12-month prospective study. J Clin Endocrinol Metab. 2002 Mar;87(3):1088-93

Hypercholesterolemia: the improvement with GH treatment

94.   Abrahamsen B, Nielsen TL, Hangaard J, Gregersen G, Vahl N, Korsholm L, Hansen TB, Andersen M, Hagen C. Dose-, IGF-I- and sex-dependent changes in lipid profile and body composition during GH replacement therapy in adult onset GH deficiency. Eur J Endocrinol. 2004 May;150(5):671-9
95.   Elgzyri T, Castenfors J, Hagg E, Backman C, Thoren M, Bramnert M. The effects of GH replacement therapy on cardiac morphology and function, exercise capacity and serum lipids in elderly patients with GH deficiency. Clin Endocrinol (Oxf). 2004 Jul;61(1):113-22
96.   Jallad RS, Liberman B, Vianna CB, Vieira ML, Ramires JA, Knoepfelmacher M.Effects of growth hormone replacement therapy on metabolic and cardiac parameters, in adult patients with childhood-onset growth hormone deficiency. Growth Horm IGF Res. 2003 Apr-Jun;13(2-3):81-8
97.   Olsovska V, Siprova H, Beranek M, Soska V. The influence of long-term growth hormone replacement therapy on body composition, bone tissue and some metabolic parameters in adults with growth hormone deficiency. Vnitr Lek. 2005 Dec;51(12):1356-64 *("a decrease of total and LDL cholesterol occurred already after a half of the year of the treatment (p < 0.05), changes were significant also in further four years. HDL cholesterol levels have had a progressive tendency, but they were not statistically significant")*

Homocysteinemia: the improvement with GH treatment

98.   Sesmilo G, Biller BM, Llevadot J, Hayden D, Hanson G, Rifai N, Klibanski A. Effects of growth hormone (GH) administration on homocyst(e)ine levels in men with GH deficiency: a randomized controlled trial. J Clin Endocrinol Metab. 2001 Apr;86(4):1518-24

Atherosclerosis: the association with lower GH and/or IGF-1 levels

99.   Capaldo B, Patti L, Oliviero U, Longobardi S, Pardo F, Vitale F, Fazio S, Di Rella F, Biondi B, Lombardi G, Sacca L. Increased arterial intima-media thickness in childhood-onset growth hormone deficiency. J Clin Endocrinol Metab. 1997 May;82(5):1378-81
100.   Markussis V, Beshyah SA, Fisher C, Sharp P, Nicolaides AN, Johnston DG. Detection of premature atherosclerosis by high-resolution ultrasonography in

symptom-free hypopituitary adults. Lancet. 1992;34():1188-1192.

101. Pfeifer M, Verhovec R, Zizek B, Prezelj J, Poredos P, Clayton RN. Growth hormone (GH) treatment reverses early atherosclerotic changes in GH-deficient adults. J Clin Endocrinol Metab. 1999 Feb;84(2):453-7

Atherosclerosis: the improvement with GH treatment

102. Pfeifer M, Verhovec R, Zizek B, Prezelj J, Poredos P, Clayton RN. Growth hormone (GH) treatment reverses early atherosclerotic changes in GH-deficient adults. J Clin Endocrinol Metab. 1999 Feb;84(2):453-7

103. Irving RJ, Carson MN, Webb DJ, Walker BR. Peripheral vascular structure and function in men with contrasting GH levels. J Clin Endocrinol Metab. 2002 Jul;87(7):3309-14

104. Borson-Chazot F, Serusclat A, Kalfallah Y, Ducottet X, Sassolas G, Bernard S, Labrousse F, Pastene J, Sassolas A, Roux Y, Berthezene F. Decrease in carotid intima-media thickness after one year growth hormone (GH) treatment in adults with GH deficiency. J Clin Endocrinol Metab. 1999 Apr;84(4):1329-33.

105. Soares DV, Spina LD, de Lima Oliveira Brasil RR, da Silva EM, Lobo PM, Salles E, Coeli CM, Conceicao FL, Vaisman M. Carotid artery intima-media thickness and lipid profile in adults with growth hormone deficiency after long-term growth hormone replacement. Metabolism. 2005 Mar;54(3):321

Arterial hypertension: the association with lower GH and/or IGF-1 levels

106. Landin-Wilhelmsen K, Wilhelmsen L, Lappas G, Rosen T, Lundstedt G, Lundberg PA, Bengtssopn BA. Serum insulin-like growth factor 1 in a random population sample of men and women: relation to age, sex, smoking habits, coffee consumption and physical activity, blood pressure and concentrations of plasma lipids, fibrinogen, parathyroid hormone and osteocalcin. Clin Endocrinol (Oxf). 1994 Sep;41(3):351-7

Arterial hypertension: the improvement with GH treatment

107. Caidahl K, Eden S, Bengtsson BA. Cardiovascular and renal effects of growth hormone. Clin Endocrinol (Oxf). 1994 Mar;40(3):393-400

Coronary heart disease: the association with lower GH and/or IGF-1 levels

108. Conti E, Andreotti F, Sciahbasi A, Riccardi P, Marra G, Menini E, Ghirlanda G, Maseri A. Markedly reduced insulin-like growth factor-1 in the acute phase of myocardial infarction. J Am Coll Cardiol. 2001 Jul;38(1):26-32

Coronary heart disease: the improvement with GH treatment

109. Castagnino HE, Lago N, Centrella JM, Calligaris SD, Farina S, Sarchi MI, Cardinali DP. Cytoprotection by melatonin and growth hormone in early rat myocardial infarction as revealed by Feulgen DNA staining. Neuroendocrinol Lett; 2002 Oct-Dec;23(5/6):391-395

Stroke and other cerebrovascular disorders: the association with GH and/or IGF-1 levels

110. Rudman D, Nagraj HS, Mattson DE, Jackson DL, Rudman IW, Boswell J, Pucci DC. Hyposomatomedinemia in the men of a Veterans Administration Nursing Home:prevalence and correlates.Gerontology. 1987;33(5):307-14

Obesity: the association with lower GH and/or IGF-1 levels

111. Beshyah SA, Freemantle C, Thomas E, Rutherford O, Page B, Murphy M, Johnston DG. Abnormal body composition and reduced bone mass in growth hormone deficient hypopituitary adults. Clin Endocrinol (Oxf) 1995 Feb;42(2):179-89

112. Attanasio AF, Bates PC, Ho KK, Webb SM, Ross RJ, Strasburger CJ, Bouillon R, Crowe B, Selander K, Valle D, Lamberts SW; Hypoptiuitary Control and Complications Study International Advisory Board. Human growth hormone replacement in adult hypopituitary patients: long-term effects on body composition and lipid status--3-year results from the HypoCCS Database. J Clin Endocrinol Metab. 2002 Apr;87(4):1600-6

113. Stouthart PJ, de Ridder CM, Rekers-Mombarg LT, van der Waal HA. Changes in body composition during 12 months after discontinuation of growth hormone therapy in young adults with growth hormone deficiency from childhood. J Pediatr Endocrinol Metab. 1999 Apr;12 Suppl 1:335-8

114. Biller BM, Sesmilo G, Baum HB, Hayden D, Schoenfeld D, Klibanski A. Withdrawal of long-term physiological growth hormone (GH) administration: differential effects on bone density and body composition in men withadult-onset GH deficiency. J Clin Endocrinol Metab. 2000 Mar;85(3):970-6

115. Kohno H, Ueyama N, Honda S. Unfavourable impact of growth hormone (GH) discontinuation on body composition and cholesterol profiles after the completion of height growth in GH-deficient young adults. Diabetes Obes Metab. 1999 Sep;1(5):293-6

116. Kuromaru R, Kohno H, Ueyama N, Hassan HM, Honda S, Hara T. Long-term prospective study of body composition and lipid profiles during and after growth hormone (GH) treatment in children with GH deficiency: gender-specific metabolic effects. J Clin Endocrinol Metab. 1998 Nov;83(11):3890-

6Vahl N, Juul A, Jorgensen JO, Orskov H, Skakkebaek NE, Christiansen JS. Continuation of growth hormone (GH) replacement in GH-deficient patients during transition from childhood to adulthood: a two-year placebo-controlled study. J Clin Endocrinol Metab. 2000 May;85(5):1874-81

117.	Norrelund H, Vahl N, Juul A, Moller N, Alberti KG, Skakkebaek NE, Christiansen JS, Jorgensen JO. Continuation of growth hormone (GH) therapy in GH-deficient patients during transition from childhood to adulthood: impact on insulin sensitivity and substrate metabolism. J Clin Endocrinol Metab. 2000 May;85(5):1912-7

118.	Johannsson G. What happens when growth hormone is discontinued at completion of growth? Metabolic aspects. J Pediatr Endocrinol Metab. 2000;13 Suppl 6:1321-6

Obesity: the improvement with GH treatment

119.	Rudman D, Feller AG, Nagraj HS, Gergans GA, Lalitha PY, Goldberg AF, Schlenker RA, Cohn L, Rudman IW, Mattson DE. Effects of human growth hormone in men over 60 years old. N Engl J Med. 1990 Jul 5;323(1):1-6

120.	Rudman D, Feller AG, Cohn L, Shetty KR, Rudman IW, Draper MW. Effects of human growth hormone on body composition in elderly men. Horm Res 1991;36 Suppl 1:73-81

121.	Bengtsson BA, Eden S, Lonn L, Kvist H, Stokland A, Lindstedt G, Bosaeus I, Tolli J, Sjostrom L, Isaksson OG. Treatment of adults with growth hormone (GH) deficiency with recombinant human GH. J Clin Endocrinol Metab. 1993 Feb;76(2):309-17

122.	Munzer T, Harman SM, Hees P, Shapiro E, Christmas C, Bellantoni MF, Stevens TE, O'Connor KG, Pabst KM, St Clair C, Sorkin JD, Blackman MR. Effects of GH and/or sex steroid administration on abdominal subcutaneous and visceral fat in healthy aged women and men. J Clin Endocrinol Metab. 2001 Aug;86(8):3604-10

123.	Rodriguez-Arnao J, Jabbar A, Fulcher K, Besser GM, Ross RJ. Effects of growth hormone replacement on physical performance and body composition in GH deficient adults. Clin Endocrinol (Oxf). 1999 Jul;51(1):53-60

124.	Soares CN, Musolino NR, Cunha Neto M, Caires MA, Rosenthal MC, Camargo CP, Bronstein MD. Impact of recombinant human growth hormone (RH-GH) treatment on psychiatric, neuropsychological and clinical profiles of GH deficient adults. A placebo-controlled trial. Arq Neuropsiquiatr. 1999 Jun;57(2A):182-9

125.	Fernholm R, Bramnert M, Hagg E, Hilding A, Baylink DJ, Mohan S, Thoren M. Growth hormone replacement therapy improves body composition and increases bone metabolism in elderly patients with pituitary disease. J Clin Endocrinol Metab. 2000 Nov;85(11):4104-12

126. Attanasio AF, Lamberts SW, Matranga AM, Birkett MA, Bates PC, Valk NK, Hilsted J, Bengtsson BA, Strasburger CJ. Adult growth hormone (GH)-deficient patients demonstrate heterogeneity between childhood onset and adult onset before and during human GH treatment. Adult Growth Hormone Deficiency Study Group. J Clin Endocrinol Metab. 1997 Jan;82(1):82-8

127. Beshyah SA, Freemantle C, Shahi M, Anyaoku V, Merson S, Lynch S, Skinner E, Sharp P, Foale R, Johnston DG. Replacement treatment with biosynthetic human growth hormone in growth hormone-deficient hypopituitary adults Clin Endocrinol (Oxf). 1995 Jan;42(1):73-84

128. Moorkens G, Wynants H, Abs R. Effect of growth hormone treatment in patients with chronic fatigue syndrome: a preliminary study. Growth Horm IGF Res. 1998 Apr;8 Suppl B:131-3

129. Lo JC, Mulligan K, Noor MA, Schwarz JM, Halvorsen RA, Grunfeld C, Schambelan M. The effects of recombinant human growth hormone on body composition and glucose metabolism in HIV-infected patients with fat accumulation. J Clin Endocrinol Metab. 2001 Aug;86(8):3480-7

130. Christ ER, Cummings MH, Albany E, Umpleby AM, Lumb PJ, Wierzbicki AS, Naoumova RP, Boroujerdi MA, Sonksen PH, Russell-Jones DL. Effects of growth hormone (GH) replacement therapy on very low density lipoprotein apolipoprotein B100 kinetics in patients with adult GH deficiency: a stable isotope study. J Clin Endocrinol Metab. 1999 Jan;84(1):307-16

131. Florkowski CM, Collier GR, Zimmet PZ, Livesey JH, Espiner EA, Donald RA. Low-dose growth hormone replacement lowers plasma leptin and fat stores without affecting body mass index in adults with growth hormone deficiency. Clin Endocrinol (Oxf). 1996 Dec;45(6):769-73

132. Ezzat S, Fear S, Gaillard RC, Gayle C, Landy H, Marcovitz S, Mattioni T, Nussey S, Rees A, Svanberg E. Gender-specific responses of lean body composition and non-gender-specific cardiac function improvement after GH replacement in GH-deficient adults. J Clin Endocrinol Metab. 2002 Jun;87(6):2725-33

133. Weaver JU, Monson JP, Noonan K, John WG, Edwards A, Evans KA, Cunningham J. The effect of low dose recombinant human growth hormone replacement on regional fat distribution, insulin sensitivity, and cardiovascular risk factors in hypopituitary adults. J Clin Endocrinol Metab. 1995 Jan;80(1):153-9

134. Vahl N, Jorgensen JO, Hansen TB, Klausen IB, Jurik AG, Hagen C, Christiansen JS. The favourable effects of growth hormone (GH) substitution on hypercholesterolaemia in GH-deficient adults are not associated with concomitant reductions in adiposity. A 12 month placebo-controlled study. Int J Obes Relat Metab Disord. 1998 Jun;22(6):529-36

135. Hansen TB, Gram J, Jensen PB, Kristiansen JH, Ekelund B, Christiansen JS, Pedersen FB. Influence of growth hormone on whole body and regional

soft tissue composition in adult patients on hemodialysis. A double-blind, randomized, placebo-controlled study. Clin Nephrol; 2000 Feb;53(2):99-107

136. Fisker S, Vahl N, Hansen TB, Jorgensen JO, Hagen C, Orskov H, Christiansen JS. Growth hormone (GH) substitution for one year normalizes elevated GH-binding protein levels in GH-deficient adults secondary to a reduction in body fat. A placebo-controlled trial. Growth Horm IGF Res. 1998 Apr;8(2):105-

137. Baum HB, Biller BM, Finkelstein JS, Cannistraro KB, Oppenhein DS, Schoenfeld DA, Michel TH, Wittink H, Klibanski A. Effects of physiologic growth hormone therapy on bone density and body composition in patients with adult-onset growth hormone deficiency. A randomized, placebo-controlled trial. Ann Intern Med. 1996 Dec 1;125(11):883-90

138. Burman P, Johansson AG, Siegbahn A, Vessby B, Karlsson FA. Growth hormone (GH)-deficient men are more responsive to GH replacement therapy than women. J Clin Endocrinol Metab. 1997 Feb;82(2):550-5

139. Schambelan M, Mulligan K, Grunfeld C, Daar ES, LaMarca A, Kotler DP, Wang J, Bozzette SA, Breitmeyer JB. Recombinant human growth hormone in patients with HIV-associated wasting. A randomized, placebo-controlled trial. Serostim Study Group. Ann Intern Med. 1996 Dec 1;125(11):873-82

140. Lee PD, Pivarnik JM, Bukar JG, Muurahainen N, Berry PS, Skolnik PR, Nerad JL, Kudsk KA, Jackson L, Ellis KJ, Gesundheit N. A randomized, placebo-controlled trial of combined insulin-like growth factor I and low dose growth hormone therapy for wasting associated with human immunodeficiency virus infection. J Clin Endocrinol Metab. 1996 Aug;81(8):2968-75

141. Toogood AA, Shalet SM.Growth hormone replacement therapy in the elderly with hypothalamic-pituitary disease: a dose-finding study. J Clin Endocrinol Metab. 1999 Jan;84(1):131-6

Diabetes: the association with lower GH and/or IGF-1 levels

142. Nam SY, Kim KR, Cha BS, Song YD, Lim SK, Lee HC, Huh KB. Low-dose growth hormone treatment combined with diet restriction decreases insulin resistance by reducing visceral fat and increasing muscle mass in obese type 2 diabetic patients. Int J Obes Relat Metab Disord. 2001 Aug;25(8):1101-7

Diabetes: the improvement with GH treatment

143. Gotherstrom G, Svensson J, Koranyi J, Alpsten M, Bosaeus I, Bengtsson B, Johannsson G. A prospective study of 5 years of GH replacement therapy in GH-deficient adults: sustained effects on body composition, bone mass, and metabolic indices. J Clin Endocrinol Metab. 2001 Oct;86(10):4657-65

144. Svensson J, Fowelin J, Landin K, Bengtsson BA, Johansson JO. Effects of

seven years of GH-replacement therapy on insulin sensitivity in GH-deficient adults. J Clin Endocrinol Metab. 2002 May;87(5):2121-7

145. Clayton KL, Holly JM, Carlsson LM, Jones J, Cheetham TD, Taylor AM, Dunger DB. Loss of the normal relationships between growth hormone, growth hormone-binding protein and insulin-like growth factor-I in adolescents with insulin-dependent diabetes mellitus. Clin Endocrinol (Oxf). 1994 Oct;41(4):517-24

146. Yuen KC, Frystyk J, White DK, Twickler TB, Koppeschaar HP, Harris PE, Fryklund L, Murgatroyd PR, Dunger DB. Improvement in insulin sensitivity without concomitant changes in body composition and cardiovascular risk markers following fixed administration of a very low growth hormone (GH) dose in adults with severe GH deficiency. Clin Endocrinol (Oxf). 2005 Oct;63(4):428-36

Rheumatism: the association with lower GH and/or IGF-1 levels

147. Neidel J. Changes in systemic levels of insulin-like growth factors and their binding proteins in patients with rheumatoid arthritis. Clin Exp Rheumatol. 2001 Jan-Feb;19(1):81-4

148. Leal-Cerro A, Povedano J, Astorga R, Gonzalez M, Silva H, Garcia-Pesquera F, Casanueva FF, Dieguez C. The growth hormone (GH)-releasing hormone-GH-insulin-like growth factor-1 axis in patients with fibromyalgia syndrome. J Clin Endocrinol Metab. 1999 Sep;84(9):3378-81

149. Bagge E, Bengtsson BA, Carlsson L, Carlsson J. Low growth hormone secretion in patients with fibromyalgia--a preliminary report on 10 patients and 10 controls. J Rheumatol. 1998 Jan;25(1):145-8

Rheumatism: the improvement with GH treatment

150. Bennett RM, Clark SC, Walczyk J. A randomized, double-blind, placebo-controlled study of growth hormone in the treatment of fibromyalgia. Am J Med. 1998 Mar;104(3):227-31

151. Bennett R. Growth hormone in musculoskeletal pain states. Curr Pain Headache Rep. 2005 Oct;9(5):331-8

Osteoporosis: the association with lower GH and/or IGF-1 levels

152. Foldes J, Lakatos P, Zsadanyi J, Horvath C. Decreased serum IGF-I and dehydroepiandrosterone sulphate may be risk factors for the development of reduced bone mass in postmenopausal women with endogenous subclinical hyperthyroidism. Eur J Endocrinol. 1997 Mar;136(3):277-81

153. Monson JP, Abs R, Bengtsson BA, Bennmarker H, Feldt-Rasmussen U,

Hernberg-Stahl E, Thoren M, Westberg B, Wilton P, Wuster C. Growth hormone deficiency and replacement in elderly hypopituitary adults. KIMS Study Group and the KIMS International Board. Pharmacia and Upjohn International Metabolic Database. Clin Endocrinol (Oxf). 2000 Sep;53(3):281-9

154. Longobardi S, Di Rella F, Pivonello R, Di Somma C, Klain M, Maurelli L, Scarpa R, Colao A, Merola B, Lombardi G. Effects of two years of growth hormone (GH) replacement therapy on bone metabolism and mineral density in childhood and adulthood onset GH deficient patients. J Endocrinol Invest. 1999 May;22(5):333-9

155. Beckers V, Milet J, Legros JJ. Prolonged treatment with recombined growth hormone improves bone measures: study of body composition in 21 deficient adults on treatment. Ann Endocrinol (Paris). 2001 Dec;62(6):507-15

156. Gomez JM, Gomez N, Fiter J, Soler J. Effects of long-term treatment with GH in the bone mineral density of adults with hypopituitarism and GH deficiency and after discontinuation of GH replacement. Horm Metab Res. 2000 Feb;32(2):66-70

157. Kaufman JM, Taelman P, Vermeulen A, Vandeweghe M. Bone mineral status in growth hormone-deficient males with isolated and multiple pituitary deficiencies of childhood onset. J Clin Endocrinol Metab. 1992 Jan;74(1):118-23

158. Calo L, Castrignano R, Davis PA, Carraro G, Pagnin E, Giannini S, Semplicini A, D'Angelo A. Role of insulin-like growth factor-I in primary osteoporosis: a correlative study. J Endocrinol Invest. 2000 Apr;23(4):223-7

159. Colao A, Di Somma C, Pivonello R, Loche S, Aimaretti G, Cerbone G, Faggiano A, Corneli G, Ghigo E, Lombardi G. Bone loss is correlated to the severity of growth hormone deficiency in adult patients with hypopituitarism. J Clin Endocrinol Metab. 1999 Jun;84(6):1919-24

160. Nakaoka D, Sugimoto T, Kaji H, Kanzawa M, Yano S, Yamauchi M, Sugishita T, Chihara K. Determinants of bone mineral density and spinal fracture risk in postmenopausal Japanese women. Osteoporos Int. 2001;12(7):548-54

161. Rico H, Del Rio A, Vila T, Patino R, Carrera F, Espinos D. The role of growth hormone in the pathogenesis of postmenopausal osteoporosis. Arch Intern Med. 1979 Nov;139(11):1263-5

162. Ljunghall S, Johansson AG, Burman P, Kampe O, Lindh E, Karlsson FA. Low plasma levels of insulin-like growth factor 1 (IGF-1) in male patients with idiopathic osteoporosis. J Intern Med. 1992 Jul;232(1):59-64

Osteoporosis: the improvement with GH treatment

163. ter Maaten JC, de Boer H, Kamp O, Stuurman L, van der Veen EA. Long-term effects of growth hormone (GH) replacement in men with childhood-

onset GH deficiency. J Clin Endocrinol Metab. 1999 Jul;84(7):2373-80

164. Gomez JM, Gomez N, Fiter J, Soler J. Effects of long-term treatment with GH in the bone mineral density of adults with hypopituitarism and GH deficiency and after discontinuation of GH replacement. Horm Metab Res. 2000 Feb;32(2):66-70

165. Baum HB, Biller BM, Finkelstein JS, Cannistraro KB, Oppenhein DS, Schoenfeld DA, Michel TH, Wittink H, Klibanski A. Effects of physiologic growth hormone therapy on bone density and body composition in patients with adult-onset growth hormone deficiency. A randomized, placebo-controlled trial. Ann Intern Med. 1996 Dec 1;125(11):883-90

166. Valimaki MJ, Salmela PI, Salmi J, Viikari J, Kataja M, Turunen H, Soppi E. Effects of 42 months of GH treatment on bone mineral density and bone turnover in GH-deficient adults. Eur J Endocrinol 1999 Jun;140(6):545-54

167. Vandeweghe M, Taelman P, Kaufman JM.Short and long-term effects of growth hormone treatment on bone turnover and bone mineral content in adult growth hormone-deficient males. Clin Endocrinol (Oxf). 1993 Oct;39(4):409-15

168. Clanget C, Seck T, Hinke V, Wuster C, Ziegler R, Pfeilschifter J. Effects of 6 years of growth hormone (GH) treatment on bone mineral density in GH-deficient adults. Clin Endocrinol (Oxf). 2001 Jul;55(1):93-9

169. Beshyah SA, Thomas E, Kyd P, Sharp P, Fairney A, Johnston DG. The effect of growth hormone replacement therapy in hypopituitary adults on calcium and bone metabolism. Clin Endocrinol (Oxf). 1994 Mar;40(3):383-91

170. Biller BM, Sesmilo G, Baum HB, Hayden D, Schoenfeld D, Klibanski A.Withdrawal of long-term physiological growth hormone (GH) administration: differential effects on bone density and body composition in men with adult-onset GH deficiency. J Clin Endocrinol Metab 2000 Mar;85(3):970-6

171. Benbassat CA, Wass rman M, Laron Z. Changes in bone mineral density after discontinuation and early reinstitution of growth hormone (GH) in patients with childhood-onset GH deficiency. Growth Horm IGF Res. 1999 Oct;9(5):290-5

172. Sartorio A, Ortolani S, Galbiati E, Conte G, Vangeli V, Arosio M, Porretti S, Faglia. Effects of 12-month GH treatment on bone metabolism and bone mineral density in adults with adult-onset GH deficiency. J Endocrinol Invest. 2001 Apr;24(4):224-30

173. Finkenstedt G, Gasser RW, Hofle G, Watfah C, Fridrich L. Effects of growth hormone (GH) replacement on bone metabolism and mineral density in adult onset of GH deficiency: results of a double-blind placebo- controlled study with open follow-up. Eur J Endocrinol. 1997 Mar;136(3):282-9

174. Erdtsieck RJ, Pols HA, Valk NK, Van OBM, Lamberts SW, Mulder P, Birkenhager JC. Treatment of post-menopausal osteoporosis with a

combination of growth hormone and pamidronate:a placebo controlled trial. Clin Endocrinol (Oxf). 1995;43:557-565

Infections and lower immunity: the association with low growth hormone/IGF-1 levels

175.   Manfredi R, Tumietto F, Azzaroli L, Zucchini A, Chiodo F, Manfredi G. Growth hormone (GH) and the immune system: impaired phagocytic function in children with idiopathic GH deficiency is corrected by treatment with biosynthetic GH. J Pediatr Endocrinol. 1994 Jul-Sep;7(3):245-51
176.   Mynarcik DC, Frost RA, Lang CH, DeCristofaro K, McNurlan MA, Garlick PJ, Steigbigel RT, Fuhrer J, Ahnn S, Gelato MC. Insulin-like growth factor system in patients with HIV infection: effect of exogenous growth hormone administration. J Acquir Immune Defic Syndr. 1999 Sep 1;22(1):49-55
177.   Panamonta O, Kosalaraksa P, Thinkhamrop B, Kirdpon W, Ingchanin C, Lumbiganon P. Endocrine function in thai children infected with human immunodeficiency virus. J Pediatr Endocrinol Metab. 2004 Jan;17(1):33-40
178.   Gupta KL, Shetty KR, Agre JC, Cuisinier MC, Rudman IW, Rudman D. Human growth hormone effect on serum IGF-I and muscle function in poliomyelitisn survivors. Arch Phys Med Rehabil. 1994 Aug;75(8):889-94

Infections and lower immunity: The improvement with GH treatment

179.   Knyszynski A, Adler-Kunin S, Globerson A. Effects of growth hormone on thymocyte development from progenitor cells in the bone marrow. Brain Behav Immun. 1992 Dec;6(4):327-40
180.   Beschorner WE, Divic J, Pulido H, Yao X, Kenworthy P, Bruce G. Enhancement of thymic recovery after cyclosporine by recombinant human growth hormone and insulin-like growth factor I. Transplantation. 1991 Nov;52(5):879-84
181.   Murphy WJ, Durum SK, Longo DL. Role of neuroendocrine hormones in murine T cell development. Growth hormone exerts thymopoietic effects in vivo. J Immunol. 1992 Dec 15;149(12):3851-7
182.   Kappel M, Hansen MB, Diamant M, Jorgensen JO, Gyhrs A, Pedersen BK. Effects of an acute bolus growth hormone infusion on the human immune system. Horm Metab Res. 1993 Nov;25(11):579-85)
183.   Kudsk KA, Mowatt-Larssen C, Bukar J, Fabian T, Oellerich S, Dent DL, Brown R. Effect of recombinant human insulin-like growth factor I and early total parenteral nutrition on immune depression following severe head injury. Arch Surg. 1994 Jan;129(1):66-70
184.   Manfredi R, Tumietto F, Azzaroli L, Zucchini A, Chiodo F, Manfredi G. Growth hormone (GH) and the immune system: impaired phagocytic

function in children with idiopathic GH deficiency is corrected by treatment with biosynthetic GH. J Pediatr Endocrinol. 1994 Jul-Sep;7(3):245-51

185. Jardieu P, Clark R, Mortensen D, Dorshkind K. In vivo administration of insulin-like growth factor-I stimulates primary B lymphopoiesis and enhances lymphocyte recovery after bone marrow transplantation. J Immunol. 1994 May 1;152(9):4320-7

186. Vara-Thorbeck R, Guerrero JA, Rosell J, Ruiz-Requena E, Capitan JM. Exogenous growth hormone: effects on the catabolic response to surgically produced acute stress and on postoperative immune function. World J Surg. 1993 Jul-Aug;17(4):530-7

187. Peake GT, Mackinnon LT, Sibbitt WL Jr, Kraner JC. Exogenous growth hormone treatment alters body composition and increases natural killer cell activity in women with impaired endogenous growth hormone secretion. Metabolism. 1987 Dec;36(12):1115-7

188. Crist DM, Kraner JC. Supplemental growth hormone increases the tumor cytotoxic activity of natural killer cells in healthy adults with normal growth hormone secretion. Metabolism. 1990 Dec;39(12):1320-4

Cancer: the association with lower GH and/or IGF-1 levels

189. Woodson K, Tangrea JA, Pollak M, Copeland TD, Taylor PR, Virtamo J, Albanes D. Serum IGF-1: tumor marker or etiologic factor? A prospective study of prostate cancer among Finnish men. Cancer Res. 2003 Jul 15;63(14):3991-4

190. Baffa R, Reiss K, El-Gabry EA, Sedor J, Moy ML, Shupp-Byrne D, Strup SE, Hauck WW, Baserga R, Gomella LG. Low serum insulin-like growth factor 1 (IGF-1): a significant association with prostate cancer. Tech Urol. 2000 Sep;6(3):236-9

191. Finne P, Auvinen A, Koistinen H, Zhang WM, Maattanen L, Rannikko S, Tammela T, Seppala M, Hakama M, Stenman UH. Insulin-like growth factor I is not a useful marker of prostate cancer in men with elevated levels of prostate-specific antigen. J Clin Endocrinol Metab. 2000 Aug;85(8):2744-7

192. Chokkalingam AP, Pollak M, Fillmore CM, Gao YT, Stanczyk FZ, Deng J, Sesterhenn IA, Mostofi FK, Fears TR, Madigan MP, Ziegler RG, Fraumeni JF Jr, Hsing AW. Insulin-like growth factors and prostate cancer: a population-based case-control study in China. Cancer Epidemiol Biomarkers Prev. 2001 May;10(5):421-7

193. Colombo F, Iannotta F, Fachinetti A, Giuliani F, Cornaggia M, Finzi G, Mantero G, Fraschini F, Malesci A, Bersani M, et al. [Changes in hormonal and biochemical parameters in gastric adenocarcinoma] Minerva Endocrinol. 1991 Jul-Sep;16(3):127-39

Cancer: opposed by GH treatment?

194.   Torosian MH. Growth hormone and prostate cancer growth and metastasis in tumor-bearing animals. J Pediatr Endocrinol. 1993 Jan-Mar;6(1):93-7

195.   Ng EH, Rock CS, Lazarus DD, Stiaino-Coico L, Moldawer LL, Lowry SF. Insulin-like growth factor I preserves host lean tissue mass in cancer cachexia. Am J Physiol. 1992 Mar;262(3 Pt 2):R426-31

196.   Bartlett DL, Charland S, Torosian MH. Growth hormone, insulin, and somatostatin therapy of cancer cachexia. Cancer. 1994 Mar 1;73(5):1499-504

III) GROWTH HORMONE MAY MAKE A PERSON SURVIVE LONGER:

Longevity: the association with GH and/or IGF-1 levels

197.   Rosen T, Bengtsson BA. Premature mortality due to cardiovascular disease in hypopituitarism. Lancet. 1990 Aug 4;336(8710):285-8

198.   Besson A, Salemi S, Gallati S, Jenal A, Horn R, Mullis PS, Mullis PE.. Reduced longevity in untreated patients with isolated growth hormone deficiency. J Clin Endocrinol Metab. 2003 Aug;88(8):3664-7

199.   Bates AS, Van't Hoff W, Jones PJ , Clayton RN. The effect of hypopituitarism on life expectancy. J Clin Endocrinol Metab. 1996;81(3):1169-72

Longevity: the improvement with GH treatment

200.   Khansari DN, Gustad T. Effects of long-term, low-dose growth hormone therapy on immune function and life expectancy of mice. Mech Ageing Dev. 1991 Jan;57(1):87-100

201.   Sonntag WE, Carter CS, Ikeno Y, Ekenstedt K, Carlson CS, Loeser RF, Chakrabarty S, Lee S, Bennett C, Ingram R, Moore T, Ramsey M. Adult-onset growth hormone and insulin-like growth factor I deficiency reduces neoplastic disease, modifies age-related pathology, and increases life span. Endocrinology. 2005;146(7):2920-32

202.   Bengtsson BA, Koppeschaar HP, Abs R, Bennmarker H, Hernberg-Stahl E, Westberg B, Wilton P, Monson JP, Feldt-Rasmussen U, Wuster C. Growth hormone replacement therapy is not associated with any increase in mortality. KIMS Study Group. J Clin Endocrinol Metab. 1999;84(11):4291-2

III) ADVERSE SYMPTOMS of PERSISTING LOW GROWTH HORMONE LEVELS have been abundantly reported, as has their improvement or

disappearance with growth hormone treatment.

203. Cuneo RC, Salomon F, McGauley GA, Sonksen PH. The growth hormone deficiency syndrome in adults. Clin Endocrinol (Oxf). 1992;37:387-97

204. Christ ER, Carroll PV, Russell JDL, Sonksen PH. The consequences of growth hormone deficiency in adulthood, and the effects of growth hormone replacement. Schweiz Med Wochenschr. 1997; 127:1440-9

205. Labram EK, Wilkin TJ. Growth hormone deficiency in adults and its response to growth hormone replacement. QJM. 1995;88:391-9

206. Rosen T, Johannsson G, Johansson JO, Bengtsson BA. Consequences of growth hormone deficiency in adults and the benefits and risks of recombinant human growth hormone treatment. Horm Res. 1995;43:93-9

207. Jorgensen JO, Muller J, MollerJ, Wolthers T, Vahl N, Juul A, Skakkebaek NE, Christiansen JS. Adult growth hormone deficiency. Horm Res. 1994:42:235-241

208. Lieberman SA, Hoffman AR. Growth hormone deficiency in adulls:characteristics and response to growth hormone replacement. J Pediatr. 1996;128:S58-S60.

IV) GROWTH HORMONE TREATMENT OF PARTIAL GROWTH HORMONE DEFICIENCY

209. Hertoghe T. Growth hormone therapy in aging adults. Anti-Aging Medical Therapeutics (Eds Klatz RM & Goldman R) 1997;I:10-28

GH treatment: safety, side effects, complications

210. Monson JP. Long-term experience with GH replacement therapy: efficacy and safety. Eur J Endocrinol. 2003 Apr;148 Suppl 2:S9-14

211. Cohn L, Feller AG, Draper MW, Rudman IW, Rudman D. Carpal tunnel syndrome and gynaecomastia during growth hormone treatment of elderly men with low circulating IGF-I concentrations. Clin Endocrinol Oxf. 1993 ;39:417-25

212. Daughaday WH. The possible autocrine/paracrine and endocrine roles of insulin-like growth factors of human tumors. Endocrinology. 1990; 127:1-4

213. Ezzat S, Melmed S. Clinical review 18: Are patients with acromegaly at increased risk for neoplasia? J Clin Endocrinol Metab. 1991:72:245-9

214. Brunner JE, Johnson CC, Zafar S, Peterson EL, Brunner JF, Mellinger RC. Colon cancer and polyps in acromegaly: increased risk associated with family history of colon cancer. Clin Endocrinol (Oxf). 1990;32:65-71

215. Bengtsson BA, Ed'en S, Ernest I, Od'en A, Sjogren B. Epidemiology and

long-term survival in acromegaly: a study of 166 cases diagnosed between 1955 and 1984. Acta Med Scand. 1988; 223:327-35

216. Massa G, Vanderschueren-Lodeweyckx M, Bouillon R. Five-year follow-up of growth hormone antibodies in growth hormone deficient children treated with recombinant human growth hormone. Clin Endocrinol. 1993;38:137-42

217. Kaplan SL, August GP, Blethen SL, Brown DR, Hintz RL, Johansen A, Plotnick LP, Underwood LE, Bell JJ, Blizzard RM, Foley TP, Hopwood NJ, Kirkland RT, Rosenfeld RG, Van Wyk JJ. Clinical studies with recombinant-DNA-derived methionyl human growth hormone in growth hormone deficient children. Lancet. 1986;I:697-700

218. Milner RDG, Barnes ND, Buckler JMH, Carson DJ, Hadden DR, Hughes IA, Johnston DI, Parkin JM, Price DA, Rayner PH, Savage DCL, Savage MO, Smith CS, Swift PG

219. Pirazzoli P, Cacciari E, Mandini M, Cicognani A, Zucchini S, Sganga T, Capelli M. Follow-up anti-bodies to growth hormone in 210 growth hormone-deficient children treated with different commercial products. Acta Paediatr. 1995 ;84:1233-6

220. Malozowski S, Tanner LA, Wysowski D, Fleming GA. Growth hormone, insulin-like growth factor I, and benign intracranial hypertension. N Engi J Med. 1993;329:665-6

221. Blethen SL, Alien DB, Graves D, August G, Moshang T, Rosenfeld R. Safety of recombinant deoxyribonucleic acid-derived growth hormone: The National Cooperative Growth Study experience. J Clin Endocrinol Metab. 1996;81:1704-10

V) JUSTIFIED OR NON JUSTIFIED FEARS ON GROWTH HORMONE TREATMENT?

1) Can growth hormone treatment cause severe discomfort and side effects?

Claim: GH treatment has substantial adverse effects such as edema, etc.
Fact: Substantial adverse effects only appear at overdoses such as is the case for any other medical treatment, it is sufficient to reduce the dose to avoid them.

1.   Wuster C, Melchinger U, Eversmann T, Hensen J, Kann P, von zur Muhlen A, Ranke MB, Schmeil H, Steinkamp H, Tuschy U. Reduced incidence of side-effects of growth hormone substitution in 404 patients with hypophyseal insufficiency. Results of a multicenter indications Study. Med Klin. 1998 Oct 15;93(10):585-91

2.   Amato G, Izzo G, La Montagna G, Bellastella A. Low dose recombinant human growth hormone normalizes bone metabolism and cortical bone density and improves trabecular bone density in growth hormone deficient adults without causing adverse effects. Clin Endocrinol (Oxf). 1996 Jul;45(1):27-32 *(no adverse effects with doses of 10μg/kg/day or a mean of 500-800 μg /day)*
3.   Chihara K, Koledova E, Shimatsu A, Kato Y, Kohno H, Tanaka T, Teramoto A, Bates PC, Attanasio AF. An individualized GH dose regimen for long-term GH treatment in Japanese patients with adult GH deficiency. Eur J Endocrinol. 2005 Jul;153(1):57-65 *("The incidence of oedema and cases with high IGF-I level were less frequent under the IGF-I controlled regimen compared with those during the fixed-dose titration method")*

2) Can growth hormone treatment cause or aggravate diabetes?

Suspicion: Can GH at physiological doses cause diabetes?
Facts: GH's role is to prevent hypoglycaemia by elevating the low serum glucose levels of GH deficient subjects back to normal. It does not at physiological doses cause diabetes.

Arguments against GH use

GH is a hyperglycemic hormone

1.   Ward PS, Savage DC. Growth hormone responses to sleep, insulin hypoglycaemia and arginine infusion. Horm Res. 1985;22(1-2):7-11

Treatment of GH-deficient children: higher incidence of diabetes

2.   Cutfield WS, Wilton P, Bennmarker H, Albertsson-Wikland K, Chatelain P, Ranke MB, Price DA . Incidence of diabetes mellitus and impaired glucose tolerance in children and adolescents receiving growth-hormone treatment. : Lancet. 2000 Feb 19;355(9204):610-3 *("GH treatment did not affect the incidence of type 1 diabetes mellitus in any age group. ... the higher than expected incidence of type 2 diabetes mellitus with GH treatment may be an acceleration of the disorder in predisposed individuals. Type 2 diabetes did not resolve after GH therapy was stopped."; critics: very high GH doses are used in children; no increased incidence of type 2 diabetes has been seen in adults taking GH)*

Serum GH levels are higher in diabetes patients *(critics: yes, two times higher serum GH, but -50% low er serum IGF-1, which reflects GH activity; insulin treatment of diabetes significantly increases serum IGF-1 and lower GH)*

3. Shishko PI, Sadykova RE, Kovalev PA, Goncharov BV. Insulin-like growth factor I in patients with newly detected insulin-dependent diabetes mellitus. Probl Endokrinol (Mosk). 1992 Jan-Feb;38(1):17-9

Acromegaly is associated with an increased incidence of diabetes

4. Mercado M, Espinosa de los Monteros AL, Sosa E, Cheng S, Mendoza V, Hernandez I, Sandoval C, Guinto G, Molina M. Clinical-biochemical correlations in acromegaly at diagnosis and the real prevalence of biochemically discordant disease. Horm Res. 2004;62(6):293-9.
5. Mestron A, Webb SM, Astorga R, Benito P, Catala M, Gaztambide S, Gomez JM, Halperin I, Lucas-Morante T, Moreno B, Obiols G, de Pablos P, Paramo C, Pico A, Torres E, Varela C, Vazquez JA, Zamora J, Albareda M, Gilabert M. Epidemiology, clinical characteristics, outcome, morbidity and mortality in acromegaly based on the Spanish Acromegaly Registry (Registro Espanol de Acromegalia, REA). Eur J Endocrinol. 2004 Oct;151(4):439-46
6. Fukuda I, Hizuka N, Murakami Y, Itoh E, Yasumoto K, Sata A, Takano K. Clinical features and therapeutic outcomes of 65 patients with acromegaly at Tokyo Women's Medical University. Intern Med. 2001 Oct;40(10):987-92

Arguments for GH use:

Insulin secretion: the tonic secretion of insulin from the beta-cells depends on IGF-1

7. Kulkarni RN, Holzenberger M, Shih DQ, Ozcan U, Stoffel M, Magnuson MA, Kahn CR.   Beta-cell-specific deletion of the Igf1 receptor leads to hyperinsulinemia and glucose intolerance but does not alter beta-cell mass. Nat Genet. 2002 May;31(1):111-5

GH is an anti-hypoglycemic hormone: it neutralizes hypoglycaemia

8. Ward PS, Savage DC. Growth hormone responses to sleep, insulin hypoglycaemia and arginine infusion. Horm Res. 1985;22(1-2):7-11
9. West TE, Sonksen PH. Is the growth-hormone response to insulin due to hypoglycaemia, hyperinsulinaemia or a fall in plasma free fatty acids? Clin Endocrinol (Oxf). 1977 Oct;7(4):283-8 *(hypoglycaemia per se was the important stimulus to GH secretion and not hyperinsulinaemia or a lowering of plasma free fatty acids)*
10. Khaleeli A, Perumainar M, Spedding AV, Teale JD, Marks V. Treatment of tumour-induced hypoglycaemia with human growth hormone. J R Soc Med. 1992 May;85(5):303

IGF-1 therapy has insulin-like effects: it reduces glycaemia and serum insulin in controls and type 2 diabetic patients

11. Moses AC, Young SC, Morrow LA, O'Brien M, Clemmons DR. Recombinant human insulin-like growth factor I increases insulin sensitivity and improves glycemic control in type II diabetes. Diabetes. 1996 Jan;45(1):91-100

Diabetes: the association with lower GH and/or IGF-1 levels

12. Nam SY, Kim KR, Cha BS, Song YD, Lim SK, Lee HC, Huh KB. Low-dose growth hormone treatment combined with diet restriction decreases insulin resistance by reducing visceral fat and increasing muscle mass in obese type 2 diabetic patients. Int J Obes Relat Metab Disord. 2001 Aug;25(8):1101-7

Diabetes patients have high GH, but low IGF-1, marker of GH metabolic activity: *a lower IGF-1 in insulin-dependent diabetes pubers is associated with a higher serum glycosylated hemoglobine HbA1C)*

13. Clayton KL, Holly JM, Carlsson LM, Jones J, Cheetham TD, Taylor AM, Dunger DB. Loss of the normal relationships between growth hormone, growth hormone-binding protein and insulin-like growth factor-I in adolescents with insulin-dependent diabetes mellitus. Clin Endocrinol (Oxf). 1994 Oct;41(4):517-24

Acromegaly: GH production in acromegaly is 10 to 100 times the normal production; 10 to 300 times the doses used in GH therapy. The pituitary GH-secreting tumor in the sella turcica crushes down the production of other pituitary hormones such as ACTH, LH, FSH, TSH, creating a **polyhormonal deficit**: hypothyroidism, hypogonadism, hypocorticism, .., endocrine conditions that increase the risk of glucose intolerance and diabetes. These conditions are not found in corrective GH treatment of GH deficiency.

14. van den Berg G, Frolich M, Veldhuis JD, Roelfsema F. Growth hormone secretion in recently operated acromegalic patients. J Clin Endocrinol Metab. 1994 Dec;79(6):1706-15 *("Patients with active acromegaly ...secretion rate per 24 h was 25 times greater in female acromegalics and 100 times greater in male acromegalics than that in the controls")*
15. Lamberton RP, Jackson IM. Investigation of hypothalamic-pituitary disease. J Clin Endocrinol Metab. 1983 Nov;12(3):509-34 *("The possibility of deficiencies of the other pituitary hormones should then be addressed in patients with secretory tumours. In patients with large macroadenomas pituitary hormone deficiencies are almost invariable with GH and FSH/LH*

being the most commonly affected, followed by TSH and ACTH in that order. Basal thyroid function tests, serum oestradiol or testosterone, and basal gonodotrophins should be routinely obtained in patients with macroadenomas. Additionally, the integrity of the pituitary-adrenal axis should be determined and an overnight water deprivation test for assessment of neurohypophyseal function is also recommended.")

16.   Snyder PJ, Bigdeli H, Gardner DF, Mihailovic V, Rudenstein RS, Sterling FH, Utiger RD. Gonadal function in fifty men with untreated pituitary adenomas. J Clin Endocrinol Metab. 1979 Feb;48(2):309-14

17.   Valenta LJ, Sostrin RD, Eisenberg H, Tamkin JA, Elias AN. Diagnosis of pituitary tumors by hormone assays and computerized tomography. Am J Med. 1982 Jun;72(6):861-73

GH therapy increases the glycaemia during the first months, then reduces it when given to HIV-infected patients with fat accumulation:

18.   Lo JC, Mulligan K, Noor MA, Schwarz JM, Halvorsen RA, Grunfeld C, Schambelan M. The effects of recombinant human growth hormone on body composition and glucose metabolism in HIV-infected patients with fat accumulation. J Clin Endocrinol Metab. 2001 Aug;86(8):3480-7

GH therapy at physiological doses to type 1 diabetics: no effect on glycaemia

19.   Bright GM, Melton RW, Rogol AD, Clarke WL. The effect of exogenous growth hormone on insulin requirements during closed loop insulin delivery in insulin-dependent diabetes mellitus. Horm Metab Res. 1984 Jun;16(6):286-9

GH therapy to type 1 diabetics: increased insulin requirements, but improved control of hypoglycaemic attacks

20.   Christ ER, Simpson HL, Breen L, Sonksen PH, Russell-Jones DL, Kohner EM. The effect of growth hormone (GH) replacement therapy in adult patients with type 1 diabetes mellitus and GH deficiency. Clin Endocrinol (Oxf). 2003 Mar;58(3):309-15

Low dose GH therapy (0.10 mg/day) improves insulin sensitivity in young healthy adults

21.   Yuen KC, Frystyk J, White DK, Twickler TB, Koppeschaar HP, Harris PE, Fryklund L, Murgatroyd PR, Dunger DB. Improvement in insulin sensitivity

without concomitant changes in body composition and cardiovascular risk markers following fixed administration of a very low growth hormone (GH) dose in adults with severe GH deficiency. Clin Endocrinol (Oxf). 2005 Oct;63(4):428-36 *("The low GH dose (0.10 mg/day) decreased fasting glucose levels (P < 0.01) and enhanced insulin sensitivity (P < 0.02), the standard GH (mean dose 0.48 mg/day) did not modify insulin sensitivity")*

Diabetes: the improvement with GH treatment

22. Gotherstrom G, Svensson J, Koranyi J, Alpsten M, Bosaeus I, Bengtsson B, Johannsson G. A prospective study of 5 years of GH replacement therapy in GH-deficient adults: sustained effects on body composition, bone mass, and metabolic indices. J Clin Endocrinol Metab. 2001 Oct;86(10):4657-65
23. Svensson J, Fowelin J, Landin K, Bengtsson BA, Johansson JO. Effects of seven years of GH-replacement therapy on insulin sensitivity in GH-deficient adults. J Clin Endocrinol Metab. 2002 May;87(5):2121-7
24. Clayton KL, Holly JM, Carlsson LM, Jones J, Cheetham TD, Taylor AM, Dunger DB. Loss of the normal relationships between growth hormone, growth hormone-binding protein and insulin-like growth factor-I in adolescents with insulin-dependent diabetes mellitus. Clin Endocrinol (Oxf). 1994 Oct;41(4):517-24
25. Yuen KC, Frystyk J, White DK, Twickler TB, Koppeschaar HP, Harris PE, Fryklund L, Murgatroyd PR, Dunger DB. Improvement in insulin sensitivity without concomitant changes in body composition and cardiovascular risk markers following fixed administration of a very low growth hormone (GH) dose in adults with severe GH deficiency. Clin Endocrinol (Oxf). 2005 Oct;63(4):428-36

3) Can growth hormone treatment cause or facilitate cancer?

Claim: GH increases the risk of cancer
Facts: The epidemiological studies, which indicate an association between serum IGF-I and cancer risk, have not established causality. An increased cancer risk with GH therapy has not been proven in humans.

Arguments against GH use:

GH LEVELS: Studies with positive associations between higher serum GH and/or IGF-1 levels and an increased risk of prostate or breast cancer

Studies where a higher serum IGF-1 and/or high IGF-I to IGFBP-3 molar ratio was found associated with an increased risk of prostate cancer *(critics: the increased IGF-1 may be due to local production of IGF-1 by the tumour and may thus be a marker, and not a cause of cancer, or a bias due to nutritional fators - see further)*

1. Peng L, Tang S, Xie J, Luo T, Dai B. Quantitative analysis of IGF-1 and its application in the diagnosis of prostate cancer. Hua Xi Yi Ke Da Xue Xue Bao. 2002 Jan;33(1):137
2. Li L, Yu H, Schumacher F, Casey G, Witte JS. Relation of serum insulin-like growth factor-I (IGF-I) and IGF binding protein-3 to risk of prostate cancer (United States). Cancer Causes Control. 2003 Oct;14(8):721-6
3. Chokkalingam AP, Pollak M, Fillmore CM, Gao YT, Stanczyk FZ, Deng J, Sesterhenn IA, Mostofi FK, Fears TR, Madigan MP, Ziegler RG, Fraumeni JF Jr, Hsing AW. Insulin-like growth factors and prostate cancer: a population-based case-control study in China. Cancer Epidemiol Biomarkers Prev. 2001 May;10(5):421-7
4. Harman SM, Metter EJ, Blackman MR, Landis PK, Carter HB. Baltimore Longitudinal Study on Aging. Serum levels of IGF-I, IGF-II, IGF-BP-3, and PSA as predictors of clinical prostate cancer. J Clin Endocrinol Metab. 2000 Nov;85(11):4258-65

Studies where a higher serum GH was found associated with an increased risk of breast cancer *(critic: based on the measurement of the daytime serum GH level, which is not representative of GH 24-hour secretion)*

5. Emerman JT, Leahy M, Gout PW, Bruchovsky N. Elevated growth hormone levels in sera from breast cancer patients. Horm Metab Res. 1985 Aug;17(8):421-4

Studies where a higher serum IGF-1 or IGF-1/IGF-BP-3 ratio is found associated with an increased risk of breast cancer, in particular in women with ≥ 19 CA repeats in IGF-1 gene

6. Yu H, Li BD, Smith M, Shi R, Berkel HJ, Kato I.. Polymorphic CA repeats in the IGF-I gene and breast cancer. Breast Cancer Res Treat. 2001 Nov;70(2):117-22
7. Vadgama JV, Wu Y, Datta G, Khan H, Chillar R. Plasma insulin-like growth factor-I and serum IGF-binding protein 3 can be associated with the progression of breast cancer, and predict the risk of recurrence and the probability of survival in African-American and Hispanic women. Oncology.

1999 Nov;57(4):330-40 *(up to 7x greater breast cancer incidence in women in the highest quintile of serum IGF-1: serum IGFBP-3 ratio compared to women in the lowest quintile)*

A study where a lower serum IGF-BP-3 was found in breast cancer patients

8.   Bruning PF, Van Doorn J, Bonfrer JM, Van Noord PA, Korse CM, Linders TC, Hart AA. Insulin-like growth-factor-binding protein 3 is decreased in early-stage operable pre-menopausal breast cancer. Int J Cancer. 1995 Jul 28;62(3):266-70

A study where a higher serum IGF-1 / IGF-BP-3 was found associated with an increased colon cancer risk *(the colon cancer risk was 4 times increased only for subjects in the upper tertile of IGF-1 and lower tertile of IGF-BP-3; for other tertiles or a combination of tertiles there was: no significant association)*

9.   Ma J, Pollak MN, Giovannucci E, Chan JM, Tao Y, Hennekens CH, Stampfer MJ. Prospecftive study of colorectal cancer risk in men and plasma levels of IGF-1 and IGF-BP-3. J Natl Cancer Inst. 1999; 91: 620-5

In acromegaly, the incidence of and/or mortality from digestive cancer is increased

10. Ron E, Gridley G, Hrubec Z, Page W, Arora S, Fraumeni JF Jr. Acromegaly and gastrointestinal cancer. Cancer. 1991 Oct 15;68(8):1673-7 *(but no increase in overall cancer incidence)*
11. Orme SM, McNally RJ, Cartwright RA, Belchetz PE. Mortality and cancer incidence in acromegaly: a retrospective cohort study. United Kingdom Acromegaly Study Group. J Clin Endocrinol Metab. 1998 Aug;83(8):2730-4 *(but decreased overall incidence of cancer in acromegaly, and no increased overall cancer mortality)*

Critics: in acromegaly the GH production is 10 to 100 times the normal production, 10 to 300 times the daily doses used in GH therapy. The pituitary GH-secreting tumor in the sella turcica crushes down the production of other pituitary hormones such as ACTH, LH, FSH, TSH, creating **a polyhormonal deficit**: hypothyroidism, hypogonadism, hypocorticism, .., endocrine conditions that increase the risk of glucose intolerance and diabetes These conditions are not found in corrective GH treatment of GH deficiency.
12. van den Berg G, Frolich M, Veldhuis JD, Roelfsema F. Growth hormone secretion in recently operated acromegalic patients. J Clin Endocrinol Metab. 1994 Dec;79(6):1706-15 *("Patients with active acromegaly ...secretion rate*

per 24 h was 25 x greater in female acromegalics & 100 x greater in male acromegalics than that in the controls")

13.   Lamberton RP, Jackson IM. Investigation of hypothalamic-pituitary disease. Clin Endocrinol Metab. 1983 Nov;12(3):509-34 *("In patients with large macroadenomas pituitary hormone deficiencies are almost invariable with GH and FSH/LH being the most commonly affected, followed by TSH and ACTH in that order ")*

14.   Snyder PJ, Bigdeli H, Gardner DF, Mihailovic V, Rudenstein RS, Sterling FH, Utiger RD.   Gonadal function in fifty men with untreated pituitary adenomas. J Clin Endocrinol Metab. 1979 Feb;48(2):309-14

15.   Valenta LJ, Sostrin RD, Eisenberg H, Tamkin JA, Elias AN. Diagnosis of pituitary tumors by hormone assays and computerized tomography. Am J Med. 1982 Jun;72(6):861-73

GH TREATMENT WITH HUMAN PITUITARY GH HORMONE

A study where the use of human pituitary GH as therapy to GH-deficient patients treated during childhood and early adulthood up to 1985 was associated with an increased risk of colon cancer and overall cancer mortality *(critics: the data are based on patients having taken GH extracted from human cadavers, now only biosynthetic growth hormone is used; moreoever, the doses used in childhood are extremely high – at least seven times those used in treatment of GH-deficiency in adults)*

16.   Swerdlow AJ, Higgins CD, Adlard P, Preece MA. Risk of cancer in patients treated with human pituitary growth hormone in the UK, 1959-85: a cohort study. Lancet. 2002 Jul 27;360(9329):273-7

Neutral information and alternative explanations of a possible GH and cancer relation

Possible bias in the studies with increased prostate and breast cancer risk:_

Bias 1:_The diagnosis of cancer may be more rapidly made in patients with high IGF-1 because they may undergo more intensive scrutiny: *As raised IGF-1 may cause tissue hyperplasia, including increase in size of prostate and breast tissue, the existence of these bigger tissues and possibly of the symptoms they may cause, may lead to more intensive scrutiny, from increased rate of PSA, CEA or C1.25 measurements, to ultrasound and RX examinations, prostate or breast biopsies, and thus an increased rate of detection of very slow, asymptomatic prostate or breast cancers that would have remained undiagnosed or diagnosed much later in patients with low IGF-1. Such higher rate of cancer detection may be particularly the case* *for prostate cancer, where the number of detected prostate cancer cases is very low compared to the total number of cases found at autotopsy, and premenopausal breast cancer patients who were diagnosed within the 2 years after the first blood sample.*

17.   Cohen P, Clemmons DR, Rosenfeld RG. Does the GH-IGF axis play a role in cancer pathogenesis? Growth Horm IGF Res. 2000 Dec;10(6):297-305

Higher levels of IGF-1 or GH or acromegaly have been associated with benign prostatic hyperplasia, but not necessarily with prostate cancer

18.   Chokkalingam AP, Gao YT, Deng J, Stanczyk FZ, Sesterhenn IA, Mostofi FK, Fraumeni JF Jr, Hsing AW. Insulin-like growth factors and risk of benign prostatic hyperplasia. Prostate. 2002 Jul 1;52(2):98-105.

19.   Colao A, Marzullo P, Ferone D, Spiezia S, Cerbone G, Marino V, Di Sarno A, Merola B, Lombardi G. Prostatic hyperplasia: an unknown feature of acromegaly. J Clin Endocrinol Metab. 1998 Mar;83(3):775-9

GH and IGF-1 treament of primates can increase breast hyperplasia, not specifically breast cancer

20.   Ng ST, Zhou J, Adesanya OO, Wang J, LeRoith D, Bondy CA. Growth hormone treatment induces mammary gland hyperplasia in aging primates. Nat Med. 1997 Oct;3(10):1141-4

Bias 2: After adjustment for prostate volume, no longer significant associations between serum IGF-I and prostate cancer risk may persist *(Serum IGF-I is not useful for diagnosis of prostate cancer, but a marker of benign prostatic hyperplasia and enlargement)*

21.   Finne P, Auvinen A, Koistinen H, Zhang WM, Maattanen L, Rannikko S, Tammela T, Seppala M, Hakama M, Stenman UH. Insulin-like growth factor I is not a useful marker of prostate cancer in men with elevated levels of prostate-specific antigen. J Clin Endocrinol Metab. 2000 Aug;85(8):2744-77

Bias 3: Serum IGF-I may actually be a surrogate marker of nutritional factors *that may increase the cancer risk such as meat and milk intake (persons who eat a lot of protein, especially red meat, have higher IGF-1 levels and an increased cancer risk)*

22.   Dai Q, Xiao-ou Shu, Fan Jin, Yu-Tang Gao, Zhi-Xian Ruan, Zheng W. Consumption of Animal Foods, Cooking Methods, and Risk of Breast Cancer. Cancer Epidemiol Biom Prev. 2002;11:801-8

Link between meat, milk and/or protein intake, and prostate or breast cancer

23. Zheng W, Deitz AC, Campbell DR, Wen WQ, Cerhan JR, Sellers TA, Folsom AR, Hein DW. N-acetyltransferase 1 genetic polymorphism, cigarette smoking, well-done meat intake, and breast cancer risk. Cancer Epidemiol Biomarkers Prev. 1999 Mar;8(3):233-9

24. Norrish AE, Lynnette R. Ferguson, Mark G. Knize, James S. Felton, Susan J. Sharpe, Jackson RT. Heterocyclic Amine Content of Cooked Meat and Risk of Prostate Cancer. J Nat Cancer Inst. 1999; 91 (23):2038-44

25. Sinha R, Chow WH, Kulldorff M, Denobile J, Butler J, Garcia-Closas M, Weil R, Hoover RN, Rothman N. Well-done, grilled red meat increases the risk of colorectal adenomas. Cancer Res. 1999;59(17):4320-4

26. Butler LM, Sinha R, Millikan RC, Martin CF, Newman B, Gammon MD, Ammerman AS, Sandler RS. Heterocyclic amines, meat intake, and association with colon cancer in a population-based study. Am J Epidemiol. 2003;157(5):434-45

27. Wolk A. Diet, lifestyle and risk of prostate cancer. Acta Oncol. 2005;44(3):277-81

28. Grant WB. An ecologic study of dietary links to prostate cancer. Altern Med Review 1999; 4(3): 162-9 *(in more than 14 European countries)*

29. Cho E, Spiegelman D, Hunter DJ, Chen WY, Stampfer MJ, Colditz GA, Willett WC. Premenopausal fat intake and risk of breast cancer. J Natl Cancer Inst. 2003 Jul 16;95(14):1079-85

Red meat and milk intake is correlated with high IGF-1

30. Kaklamani VG, Linos A, Kaklamani E, Markaki I, Koumantaki Y, Mantzoros CS. Dietary fat and carbohydrates are independently associated with circulating insulin-like growth factor 1 and insulin-like growth factor-binding protein 3 concentrations in healthy adults. J Clin Oncol. 1999 Oct;17(10):3291-8

31. Larsson SC, Wolk K, Brismar K, Wolk A. Association of diet with serum insulin-like growth factor I in middle-aged and elderly men. Am J Clin Nutr. 2005 May;81(5):1163-7

32. Allen NE, Appleby PN, Davey GK, Kaaks R, Rinaldi S, Key TJ. The associations of diet with serum insulin-like growth factor I and its main binding proteins in 292 women meat-eaters, vegetarians, and vegans. Cancer Epidemiol Biomarkers Prev. 2002 Nov;11(11):1441-8

33. Hoppe C, Molgaard C, Juul A, Michaelsen KF. High intakes of skimmed milk, but not meat, increase serum IGF-I and IGFBP-3 in eight-year-old boys. Eur J Clin Nutr. 2004 Sep;58(9):1211-6

Bias 4: The increases of serum IGF-1 may be produced by the malignant tumour and constitute a consequence and not a cause as suggested in some animal studies.

34.   DiGiovanni J, Kiguchi K, Frijhoff A, Wilker E, Bol DK, Beltran L, Moats S, Ramirez A, Jorcano J, Conti C. Deregulated expression of insulin-like growth factor 1 in prostate epithelium leads to neoplasia in transgenic mice. Proc Natl Acad Sci USA. 2000 Mar 28;97(7):3455-60

35.   Kaplan PJ, Mohan S, Cohen P, Foster BA, Greenberg NM. The insulin-like growth factor axis and prostate cancer: lessons from the transgenic adenocarcinoma of mouse prostate (TRAMP) model. Cancer Res. 1999 May 1;59(9):2203-9

Bias 5: the variability of serum IGF-1 makes that if two weeks after the initial blood test another measurement of IGF-1 was done, the results of the studies would have been different (about 40° % of participants of the study would have switched from one quartile to the other)

36.   Milani D, Carmichael JD, Welkowitz J, Ferris S, Reitz RE, Danoff A, Kleinberg DL. Variability and reliability of single serum IGF-I measurements: impact on determining predictability of risk ratios in disease development. J Clin Endocrinol Metab. 2004 May;89(5):2271-4 *("If fasting serum IGF-1 is measured twice, two weeks apart, individuall differences range from -36.25 to +38.24%, while the mean value for the group of 84 shows high correlation between the two IGF-Is (r=0.922; p<0.0001) and varies much less (mean 120 at first visit) versus 115; p=0.03) in normal volunteers between the ages of 50 and 90 years. When considered in quartiles, IGF-I changed from one quartile to another in 34/84 (40.5%) of the volunteers. When the group was divided in halves, tertiles, quartiles, or quintiles there was an increasing number of subjects who changed from one subdivision to another as the number of gradations increased. These results suggest that the predictive outcomes of earlier studies that used single IGF-I samples for analysis of risk ratios according to tertiles, quartiles, or quintiles could have been different if a second IGF-I was used to establish the risk ratio.")*

No significant associations of serum levels and prostate cancer risk

No difference in plasma GH or IGF-1 between prostate cancer patients and controls

37.   Yu H, Nicar MR, Shi R, Berkel HJ, Nam R, Trachtenberg J, Diamandis EP. Levels of IGF-I and IGF BP- 2 and -3 in serial postoperative serum samples and risk of prostate cancer recurrence. Urology. 2001 Mar;57(3):471-5.

38.   Hill M, Bilek R, Safarik L, Starka L. Analysis of relations between serum levels of epitestosterone, estradiol, testosterone, IGF-1 and prostatic specific antigen in men with benign prostatic hyperplasia and carcinoma of the prostate. Physiol Res. 2000;49 Suppl 1:S113-8

39.   Kurek R, Tunn UW, Eckart O, Aumuller G, Wong J, Renneberg H. The significance of serum levels of insulin-like growth factor-1 in patients with prostate cancer. BJU Int. 2000 Jan;85(1):125-9

40.   Cutting CW, Hunt C, Nisbet JA, Bland JM, Dalgleish AG, Kirby RS. Serum insulin-like growth factor-1 is not a useful marker of prostate cancer. BJU Int. 1999 Jun;83(9):996-9

41.   Ismail HA, Pollak M, Behlouli H, Tanguay S, Begin LR, Aprikian AG. Serum insulin-like growth factor (IGF)-1 and IGF-binding protein-3 do not correlate with Gleason score or quantity of prostate cancer in biopsy samples. BJU Int. 2003 Nov;92(7):699-702

42.   Woodson K, Tangrea JA, Pollak M, Copeland TD, Taylor PR, Virtamo J, Albanes D. Serum insulin-like growth factor I: tumor marker or etiologic factor? A prospective study of prostate cancer among Finnish men. Cancer Res. 2003 Jul 15;63(14):3991-4

43.   Ismail A H, Pollak M, Behlouli H, Tanguay S, Begin LR, Aprikian AG. Insulin-like growth factor-1 and insulin-like growth factor binding protein-3 for prostate cancer detection in patients undergoing prostate biopsy. J Urol. 2002 Dec;168(6):2426-30

44.   Bubley GJ, Balk SP, Regan MM, Duggan S, Morrissey ME, Dewolf WC, Salgami E, Mantzoros C. Serum levels of insulin-like growth factor-1 and insulin-like growth factor-1 binding proteins after radical prostatectomy. J Urol. 2002 Nov;168(5):2249-52

45.   DeLellis K, Rinaldi S, Kaaks RJ, Kolonel LN, Henderson B, Le Marchand L. Dietary and lifestyle correlates of plasma insulin-like growth factor-I (IGF-I) and IGF binding protein-3 (IGFBP-3): the multiethnic cohort. Cancer Epidemiol Biomarkers Prev. 2004 Sep;13(9):1444-51.

In acromegaly, the incidence of cancer, other than possibly colon cancer, does not appear to be significantly increased; *in one study it was even significantly reduced by -14 %. Overall mortality is normal for patients with low posttreatment GH, but increased for patients with high posttreatment GH.*

46.   J. Svensson, B.-Å. Bengtsson, T. Rosén, Odén A, Johannsson G. Malignant Disease and Cardiovascular Morbidity in Hypopituitary Adults with or without

GH Replacement Therapy. J Clin Endocrinol Metab. 2004 Jul;89(7):3306-12

47.   Orme SM, McNally RJ, Cartwright RA, Belchetz PE. Mortality and cancer incidence in acromegaly: a retrospective cohort study. United Kingdom Acromegaly Study Group. J Clin Endocrinol Metab. 1998 Aug;83(8):2730-4 *("The overall cancer incidence rate was 24 % lower than that in the general population of the U.K.; the overall cancer mortality rate was not increased, but the colon cancer mortality rate was increased.")*

No difference in serum IGF-1 between breast cancer patients and controls

48.   Li BD, Khosravi MJ, Berkel HJ, Diamandi A, Dayton MA, Smith M, Yu H. Free insulin-like growth factor-I and breast cancer risk. Int J Cancer. 2001 Mar 1;91(5):736-9

49.   DeLellis K, Rinaldi S, Kaaks RJ, Kolonel LN, Henderson B, Le Marchand L. Dietary and lifestyle correlates of plasma insulin-like growth factor-I (IGF-I) and IGF binding protein-3 (IGFBP-3): the multiethnic cohort. Cancer Epidemiol Biomarkers Prev. 2004 Sep;13(9):1444-51.

GH transgenic mice with high serum IGF-1 do not develop breast, prostate, or colonic malignancies

50.   Wennbo H, Gebre-Medhin M, Gritli-Linde A, Ohlsson C, Isaksson OG, Tornell J. Activation of the prolactin receptor but not the growth hormone receptor is important for induction of mammary tumors in transgenic mice. J Clin Invest. 1997 Dec 1;100(11):2744-51

51.   Wennbo H, Tornell J. The role of prolactin and GH in breast cancer. Octogene. 2000;19:1072-6

Arguments for GH use:

Inverse (protective) associations of serum GH/IGF-1 levels and overall cancer risk

Untreated GH deficient patients have an increased overall cancer incidence (2x the normal incidence) and cancer mortality (4x)

52.   Svensson J, Bengtsson BÅ, Rosén T, Odén A, Johannsson G. Malignant disease and cardiovascular morbidity in hypopituitary adults with or without growth hormone replacement therapy. J Clin Endocrinol Metab. 2004 Jul;89(7):3306-12

A high serum IGF-1 is found associated with a lower risk of prostate cancer

53.   Finne P, Auvinen A, Koistinen H, Zhang WM, Maattanen L, Rannikko S, Tammela T, Seppala M, Hakama M, Stenman UH. Insulin-like growth factor I is not a useful marker of prostate cancer in men with elevated levels of prostate-specific antigen. J Clin Endocrinol Metab. 2000 Aug;85(8):2744-7

54.   Woodson K, Tangrea JA, Pollak M, Copeland TD, Taylor PR, Virtamo J, Albanes D. Serum IGF-1: tumor marker or etiologic factor? A prospective study of prostate cancer among Finnish men. Cancer Res. 2003;15;63(14):3991-4 *(- 48 % for men in the highest quartile of serum IGF-1)*

55.   Baffa R, Reiss K, El-Gabry EA, Sedor J, Moy ML, Shupp-Byrne D, Strup SE, Hauck WW, Baserga R, Gomella LG. Low serum insulin-like growth factor 1 (IGF-1): a significant association with prostate cancer. Tech Urol 2000 Sep;6(3):236-9

No significant association between serum IGF-1 and prostate cancer:

GH therapy increases serum IGF-BP-3, *which may protect against cancer: IGFBP-3 causes apoptosis of cancer cells and inhibits IGF action on cancer cells in vitro => Serum IGFBP-3 is in general negatively correlated with the cancer risk cancer: the higher IGF-BP-3, the lower the cancer risk*

56.   Wollmann HA, Schonau E, Blum WF, Meyer F, Kruse K, Ranke MB. Dose-dependent responses in insulin-like growth factors, insulin-like growth factor-binding protein-3 and parameters of bone metabolism to growth hormone therapy in young adults with growth hormone deficiency. Horm Res. 1995;43(6):249-56

57.   Grimberg A, Cohen P. GH & prostate cancer: guilty by association? J Endocrinol Invest. 1999;22(5 Suppl):64-73

A high serum IGF-BP-3 is associated with a reduced prostate cancer risk (-30%), and/or prostate cancer recurrence

58.   Harman SM, Metter EJ, Blackman MR, Landis PK, Carter HB. Baltimore Longitudinal Study on Aging. Serum levels of IGF-I, IGF-II, IGF-BP-3, and PSA as predictors of clinical prostate cancer. J Clin Endocrinol Metab. 2000 Nov;85(11):4258-65

Studies where GH therapy given to cancer patients reduced the cancer recurrence, and reduces the cancer mortality or increases survival time

59.   Swerdlow AJ, Reddingius RE, Higgins CD, Spoudeas HA, Phipps K, Qiao Z, Ryder WD,Brada M, Hayward RD, Brook CG, Hindmarsh PC, Shalet SM. Growth hormone treatment of children with brain tumors and risk of tumor recurrence. J Clin Endocrinol Metab. 2000 Dec;85(12):4444-9

60.   Tacke J, Bolder U, Herrmann A, Berger G, Jauch KW. Long-term risk of gastrointestinal tumor recurrence after postoperative treatment with recombinant human growth hormone. JPEN J Parenter Enteral Nutr 2000 May-Jun;24(3):140-4

Long-term GH replacement (60 months) **reduced the increased cancer risk and mortality of GH deficient patients by half**

61.   Svensson J, Bengtsson BÅ, Rosén T, Odén A, Johannsson G. Malignant disease and cardiovascular morbidity in hypopituitary adults with or without growth hormone replacement therapy. J Clin Endocrinol Metab. 2004 Jul;89(7):3306-12

GH or IGF-1 therapy to animals with cancer: may reduce the tumour incidence and/or progression

Combined GH- insulin therapy reduced the development of mammary carcinoma in female rats

62.   Bartlett DL, Charland S, Torosian MH. Growth hormone, insulin, and somatostatin therapy of cancer cachexia. Cancer. 1994 Mar 1;73(5):1499-504

GH-therapy reduced the development of lung metastases in rats with prostate cancer

63.   Torosian MH. Growth hormone and prostate cancer growth and metastasis in tumor-bearing animals. J Pediatr Endocrinol. 1993 Jan-Mar;6(1):93-7

A lower serum GH level is found in gastric cancer patients

64.   Colombo F, Iannotta F, Fachinetti A, Giuliani F, Cornaggia M, Finzi G, Mantero G, Fraschini F, Malesci A, Bersani M, et al. [Changes in hormonal and biochemical parameters in gastric adenocarcinoma] Minerva Endocrinol. 1991 Jul-Sep;16(3):127-39

GH-therapy inhibits the development of liver cancer due to carcinogens (aflatoxin B1 or N-OH-acetyl- aminofluoren) in male rats

65.   Liao D, Porsch-Hallstrom I, Gustafsson JA, Blanck A. Sex differences at the initiation stage of rat liver carcinogenesis—influence of growth hormone. Carcinogenesis. 1993 Oct;14(10):2045-9

IGF-1-therapy preserved lean mass in rats with sarcoma and cachexia

66. Ng EH, Rock CS, Lazarus DD, Stiaino-Coico L, Moldawer LL, Lowry SF. Insulin-like growth factor I preserves host lean tissue mass in cancer cachexia. Am J Physiol. 1992 Mar;262(3 Pt 2):R426-31

Conclusion on the cancer studies and GH

• **GH therapy raises both the levels of both IGF-I and IGFBP-3. IGF-BP-3** is a potent inhibitor of IGF action in breast and prostate tissues.
• **Autocrine production of IGF's and GH**, have been identified in **cancer cells and tissues**. Thus, serum IGF-I may actually be a confounding variable, serving as a marker for local prostatic IGF-I production.
• Since GH-deficient patients often have a subnormal IGF-I serum level, which normalizes on therapy, the cancer risk on **GH therapy does probably not substantially increase above that of the normal population**. On the contrary, the evidence points to a normalization of the risk.
• It seems prudent that when we treat adult GH deficiency, we should aim to maintain serum IGF-1 in the normal range.

4) CAN GROWTH HORMONE TREATMENT REDUCE THE LIFESPAN?

Claim: GH may have adverse effects on lifespan
Facts: GH treatment appears to reduce mortality, except for special mice species and humans put in extreme conditions.

Arguments against GH use

Studies where higher GH and/or IGF-1 levels were found associated with premature death

A high serum GH was associated with premature death in humans *(critics: an old fashioned technique, which lacked assay precision, was used to measure GH; the daytime serum GH were measured, which is not accurate except for acromegaly patients; serum GH does not reflect GH activity, serum IGF-1 does it, but up to a certain degree; an increased serum GH may possibly reflect increased binding of GH to increased serum GHBP and thus inactivation of GH, but the serum GHBP level was not checked in the study)*

1. Maison P, Balkau B, Simon D, Chanson P, Rosselin G, Eschwege E. Growth hormone as a risk for premature mortality in healthy subjects: data from the Paris prospective study. BMJ. 1998 Apr 11;316(7138):1132-3

Acromegaly adults have premature death only when they keep high posttreatment GH *and thus a probably continuing active growth hormone-secreting tumor that crushes down all the other pituitary cells, overall mortality is normal for patients with low posttreatment GH.*

2.   Orme SM, McNally RJ, Cartwright RA, Belchetz PE. Mortality and cancer incidence in acromegaly: a retrospective cohort study. United Kingdom Acromegaly Study Group. J Clin Endocrinol Metab. 1998 Aug;83(8):2730-4.

Mice models of genetic pituitary failure with multiple hormone deficiency (Ames and Snell mice) **and GH receptor knockout mice** (primary IGF1-deficiency) **may have a significant higher longevity** *(critics: the heterozygous IGF-I receptor knock-out mutants are special mice species, as are* Ames and Snell mice *. They react in a completely different way to GH than normal mice species. They have a 50 % decrease in IGF-1 receptors, but a 32% higher serum IGF-1; they have more glucose intolerance; are slightly smaller; the lifespan was only significantly longer in female mice (+33%), not in male mice (+16%); the results based on a shortliving species (mise) may not be necessarily true for species with a long life such as humans)*

3.   Liang H, Masoro EJ, Nelson JF, Strong R, McMahan CA, Richardson A. Genetic mouse models of extended lifespan. Exp Gerontol. 2003 Nov-Dec;38(11-12):1353-64

4.   Holzenberger M. The GH/IGF-I axis and longevity. Eur J Endocrinol. 2004 Aug;151 Suppl 1:S23-7

5.   Kulkarni RN, Holzenberger M, Shih DQ, Ozcan U, Stoffel M, Magnuson MA, Kahn CR. beta-cell-specific deletion of the Igf1 receptor leads to hyperinsulinemia and glucose intolerance but does not alter beta-cell mass. Nat Genet. 2002 May;31(1):111-5 *(lack IGF-1 receptors on beta-cells => glucose interance and less beta-cells)*

6.   Hauck SJ, Aaron JM, Wright C, Kopchick JJ, Bartke A. Antioxidant enzymes, free-radical damage, and response to paraquat in liver and kidney of long-living growth hormone receptor/binding protein gene-disrupted mice. Horm Metab Res. 2002 Sep;34(9):481-6

Can GH therapy increases mortality?

GH therapy to critically ill patients: doubles the mortality rate

7.   Takala J, Ruokonen E, Webster NR, Nielsen MS, Zandstra DF, Vundelinckx G, Hinds CJ. Increased mortality associated with growth hormone treatment

in critically ill adults. N Engl J Med. 1999 Sep 9;341(11):785-92 *(Critics on the study: the doses used were too high doses: 10 to 70 times the normal dose in very weak persons; the control group had an abnormally lower mortality rate than predicted; combined to the high mortality rates of the treatment group, the average mortality rate was very similar to that of a historical cohort; GH treatment lowers cortisol levels, which are crucial to critically ill patients)*

8.   Freeman BD, Danner RL, Banks SM, Natanson C. Safeguarding patients in clinical trials with high mortality rates. Am J Respir Crit Care Med. 2001 Jul 15;164(2):190-2

BUT: Studies where GH therapy lowered the levels of cortisol and its metabolites by 20 to 40 %, which is dangerous for critically-ill patients who desperately need cortisol for their survival

9.   Vierhapper H, Nowotny P, Waldhausl W. Treatment with growth hormone suppresses cortisol production in man. Metabolism 1998 Nov;47(11):1376-8 ;

10.   Rodriguez-Arnao J, Perry L, Besser GM, Ross RJ. Growth hormone treatment in hypopituitary GH deficient adults reduces circulating cortisol levels during hydrocortisone replacement therapy. Clin Endocrinol (Oxf). 1996 Jul;45(1):33-7

11.   Weaver JU, Thaventhiran L, Noonan K, Burrin JM, Taylor NF, Norman MR, Monson JP. The effect of growth hormone replacement on cortisol metabolism and glucocorticoid sensitivity in hypopituitary adults. Clin Endocrinol (Oxf). 1994 Nov;41(5):639-48

...and a study where patients who have poor responsive adrenals (poorly able to increase their cortisol production) and are in septic shock, die easier

12.   Rothwell PM, Udwadia ZF, Lawler PG. Cortisol response to corticotropin and survival in septic shock. Lancet. 1991 Mar 9;337(8741):582-3

.. and studies where glucocorticoid treatments considerably increased survival of critically-ill patients

survival of HIV patient from pneumonia
13.   Gagnon S, Boota AM, Fischl MA, Baier H, Kirksey OW, La Voie L. Corticosteroids as adjunctive therapy for severe Pneumocystis carinii pneumonia in the acquired immunodeficiency syndrome. A double-blind, placebo-controlled trial. N Engl J Med. 1990 Nov 22;323(21):1444-50

survival from typhus
14.   Hoffman SL, Punjabi NH, Kumala S, Moechtar MA, Pulungsih SP, Rivai AR, Rockhill RC, Woodward TE, Loedin AA. Reduction of mortality in chloramphenicol-treated severe typhoid fever by high-dose dexamethasone. N Engl J Med. 1984 Jan 12;310(2):82-8

NEUTRAL information on GH and longevity

No increased mortality in acromegaly if levels of GH are less than 2.5 ng/ml

15.   Orme SM, McNally RJ, Cartwright RA, Belchetz PE. Mortality and cancer incidence in acromegaly: a retrospective cohort study. United Kingdom Acromegaly Study Group. J Clin Endocrinol Metab. 1998 Aug;83(8):2730-4

Arguments for GH use

GH/IGF-1 LEVELS: Higher serum GH and IGF-1 levels are associated with a higher survival

Persistent GH deficiency (without GH therapy) in humans, is associated with a shorter life expectancy: increased overall and cardiovascular mortality

16.   Rosen T, Bengtsson BA. Premature mortality due to cardiovascular disease in hypopituitarism. Lancet. 1990 Aug 4;336(8710):285-8
17.   AS Bates, W Van't Hoff, PJ Jones and RN Clayton. The effect of hypopituitarism on life expectancy. J Clin Endocrin Metab. 1996 Mar;81(3):1169-72

Higher mortality in GH deficient women

18.   Svensson J, Bengtsson BÅ, Rosén T, Odén A, Johannsson G. Malignant disease and cardiovascular morbidity in hypopituitary adults with or without growth hormone replacement therapy. J Clin Endocrinol Metab. 2004 Jul;89(7):3306-12

Higher mortality in 11 GH deficient adults suffering from a genetic defect (6.7-kb spanning deletion of genomic DNA of the GH-1 gene) **that causes isolated GH deficiency (hereditary dwarfism),** *untreated men lost 21 years of life (-25% compared to the unaffected brothers) and women 34 years less (-44% versus unaffected sisters)*

19. Besson A, Salemi S, Gallati S, Jenal A, Horn R, Mullis PS, Mullis PE. Reduced longevity in untreated patients with isolated growth hormone deficiency. J Clin Endocrinol Metab. 2003;88(8):3664-7

Patients with hypopituitarism have increased overall and cardiovascular mortality; *the increased mortality from cerebrovascular disease (esp. in women) was the main contributor to the increased cardiovascular mortality*

20. Bulow B, Hagmar L, Mikoczy Z, Nordstrom CH, Erfurth EM.Increased cerebrovascular mortality in patients with hypopituitarism. Clin Endocrinol (Oxf). 1997 Jan;46(1):75-81
21. Bengtsson BA, Koppeschaar HP, Abs R, Bennmarker H, Hernberg-Stahl E, Westberg B, Wilton P, Monson JP, Feldt-Rasmussen U, Wuster C. Growth hormone replacement therapy is not associated with any increase in mortality. KIMS Study Group. J Clin Endocrinol Metab. 1999 Nov;84(11):4291-2

GH TREATMENT: Corrective GH hormone treatment increases survival

GH replacement therapy of GH deficient adults lowers the excessive mortality back to normal

22. Bengtsson BA, Koppeschaar HP, Abs R, Bennmarker H, Hernberg-Stahl E, Westberg B, Wilton P, Monson JP, Feldt-Rasmussen U, Wuster C. Growth hormone replacement therapy is not associated with any increase in mortality. KIMS Study Group. J Clin Endocrinol Metab. 1999 Nov;84(11):4291-2
23. Svensson J, Bengtsson BÅ, Rosén T, Odén A, Johannsson G. Malignant disease and cardiovascular morbidity in hypopituitary adults with or without growth hormone replacement therapy. J Clin Endocrinol Metab. 2004 Jul;89(7):3306-12

GH treatment of normal elderly mice, extended the mean and maximal life span[8-9].

24. Khansari DN, Gustad T. Effects of long-term, low-dose growth hormone therapy on immune function and life expectancy of mice. Mech Ageing Dev. 1991 Jan;57(1):87-100

GH treatment of GH deficient mice extended life span, *but lifespan of (non GH treated) mice was similar to that of normal mice.*

25. Sonntag WE, Carter CS, Ikeno Y, Ekenstedt K, Carlson CS, Loeser RF, Chakrabarty S, Lee S, Bennett C, Ingram R, Moore T, Ramsey M. Adult-onset growth hormone and insulin-like growth factor I deficiency reduces neoplastic disease modifies age-related pathology, and increases life span. Endocrinology. 2005 Jul;146(7):2920-32

Conclusion: Persistent GH deficiency reduces the life expectancy, while GH treatment of GH-deficient patients improves it. Caution should be applied when using GH treatment in critically-ill patients.

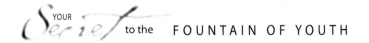

APPENDIX 2

BõKU™ Super Food

From the very young to people blessed with advanced maturity, a nutritious diet remains essential to maintain exceptional health—even when using injectable HGH. Among the best food sources, we highly recommend BõKU™ Super Food, available via the popular Web site, *BõKU™SuperFood.com*

"A little bit of BõKU will give you more nutrition than the average American gets in several days," said Dr. Brian Clement of the Hippocrates Institute.

Using only the best and healthiest-available food sources, all BõKU™ Super Food products come in either of three economical, tasty and nutritious forms: basic super foods, cleansing, and Super Bars®.

John D., a marathon runner from Santa Paula, Calif., noticed an improvement in his moods and an increase in daytime energy after eating BõKU™ Super Food for more than one month. Along with an increase in his mental alertness, John enjoyed a decrease in his food cravings plus a cleansing of his digestive system. John also started sleeping better at night.

"When I ran out of my Super Food supply, my body knew something was missing," John said, adding that he planned to use BõKU™ Super Bars while preparing for long-distance runs.

Just as important, to Allan A. of Las Vegas, "I was pleased by the reaction it produced. In short order, my mood was elevated and I had a sense of well being for the rest of the day. Also, I found myself having more energy than I had in a long time.

"With all the companies that make ridiculous and false claims to market their products, I felt compelled to tell you that your description of your BõKU™ Super Food is right on the mark," said Allan, a self-described "born skeptic" who became pleasantly surprised to discover that this food has what he calls a mild and rather nice taste.

Just as impressive, we find that BõKU™ is economical, readily absorbed by the body, and super-easy to prepare. In fact, just one tablespoon comprises an entire adult serving, with 10-ounce bottles containing 30 servings, and 30-ounce bottles with 90 servings. A child-size serving is a half tablespoon.

People consider the taste of BōKU™ as neutral and especially mild when considering the fact it's very green, dense and highly nutritious.

"Many people enjoy BōKU™ in a large glass of water, but you can blend it with almost any liquid," said Lynn M. Rollé, president and CEO of BōKU™ Super Food, the company's co-founder.

"We believe that BōKU™ is the highest quality, most nutritious dense super food on the planet, and the healthiest thing a person could ever consume," Rollé said. "Super foods are plants, vegetables, roots and fruits that are highly nutritious and health-forming."

Excellent for the entire family

During our formative and teen years, lifestyle habits and the foods we eat create the building blocks for potentially good health later during the mature phase of life.

"Our customers tell us that their children love BōKU™ Super Food blended into a glass of chocolate soy or rice milk," said Dr. B.J. Adrezin, master formulator for the company's full line of food products and its chief medical adviser.

Some people notice the benefits of BōKU™ Super Food right away, while others might take a week or more. Each person's current diet might play a key factor, along with individual health history.

However long the process takes, your body will respond with improved health and increased vitality thanks to super nutrients found in this food.

Before taking BōKU™ Super Food, some people prefer to complete a BōKU™ Super 3-day Cleanse to expel toxins and unnecessary waste from their bodies.

In creating these meals, hailed as the "world's most powerful super food formula," Dr. Adrezin combined pure organic alkalizing greens with potent quantities of unique super foods including organic maca root juice, organic goji berry, 14 organic specialty mushrooms and other foods.

"Every BōKU™ Super Food ingredient is nutrient-dense," said Adrezin, who carefully balanced every substance when creating the meals. "We use absolutely no fillers of any kind."

The finest organic ingredients comprise 95 percent of BōKU™ Super Food, while remaining ingredients come from protected, wild-crafted sources found in nature.

Adding to this benefit, the body absorbs nutrients from BōKU™ Super Food more readily than the digestive system takes in the synthetically produced nutrients from standard multi-vitamins.

"BōKU™ Super Food contains naturally occurring, non-toxic whole food vitamins and minerals that are more readily absorbed than synthetic supplements," Adrezin said. "Unfortunately, many vitamins end up passing through our bodies as waste."

By contrast, Adrezin said, direct delivery made possible by BōKU™ Super Food proves an advantage and many people feel the beneficial impact immediately.

Just as important, BōKU™ Super Food provides thousands of naturally-occurring, deeply healing phytochemicals and phytonutrients that isolated vitamins lack.

Discover ideal situations for BōKU™ Super Food

Many people who benefit from BōKU™ Super Food discover to their delight that they can enjoy such meals whenever they want. Although many individuals feel energized after absorbing the nutrients, these consumers can take comfort in knowing that the formula lacks the properties of a stimulant.

Some BōKU™ Super Food enthusiasts prefer to start out with one serving daily for the first month or so. Then, they experiment with one BōKU™ blend in the morning and another in the afternoon, or for a pre- or post-workout boost.

Adrezin says the possibility of taking too much BōKU™ Super Food is highly unlikely, since this formula contains non-toxic, natural substances. Also, keep in mind that BōKU™ is not a supplement, but instead a broad-spectrum super food.

"It is virtually impossible to overdose with BōKU™," Adrezin said. "Mega-dosing is not only safe, but encouraged. Depending on the individual and the level of toxicity, there may be adverse reactions to the cleansing benefits of BōKU™.

"As a result, common sense is the way to go. We suggest you start off with the recommended serving, and gradually increase the amount to your liking."

Keep in mind that your body absorbs the nutrients of BōKU™ Super Food faster on an empty stomach, when it's okay to drink. Also, researchers have never found any negative effects of taking BōKU™ with coffee. There's no need to refrigerate

BōKU™ Super Food, even after opening the container—but you should keep any portion chilled after mixing it with liquids in order to maintain nutritional value.

BōKU™ Super Food also has a 2- to 3-year shelf life when properly sealed and stored in its original packaging.

BōKU™ can begin cleansing and other benefits

Some users experience cleansing reactions when they first start taking BōKU™ Super Food, especially if they had eaten chemical-laden processed foods.

"BōKU™ Super Foods contain some of the most powerful and cleansing nutrients found in nature," Adrezin said. "As a result, it can initiate beneficial detoxification and cleansing reactions. For some people, this process will go on 'behind the scenes.'"

"For those who experience uncomfortable reactions such as headaches or loose bowels, simply take a smaller dose and build back up once you feel better," he said.

The extremely small number of people who suffer upset stomachs after ingesting BōKU™ can enjoy this super food after blending it into a smoothie, rather than in juice or flavored milk. Or, for a few weeks, reap the many benefits of BōKU™ Super Food after blending it in juice or milk, taking it with light meals. Other individuals use half rather than full servings, till the body adjusts.

Nursing mothers should consult their health care professionals if they have medical questions.

During the production of enzyme-active BōKU™ Super Food, the manufacturer carefully dries all ingredients at low temperatures. This maintains heat-sensitive elements including enzymes. The producer individually dries each ingredient, all enzyme active.

Some people who enjoy BōKU™ Super Food notice the good sign that their bowels are looser, having the same green color as this product. Following continued use individuals see healthy bowel movements without green.

BōKU™ Super Food is free of gluten. As standard procedure, the U.S. Customs Service x-rays deliveries passing through federal government portals like Washington,

D.C. And the law requires that officials x-ray shipments that are headed to restricted areas. Only shipments that pass through government portals get x-rayed.

So, what is BõKU™ Super Food?

The award-winning BõKU™ Super Food has a proprietary blend of the most potent, certified organic super foods in the world. To create this formula, Lynn M. Rollé and her husband, Reno Rollé, recruited Adrezin, medical director of the Center for NutriLongevity™ in Lake Oswego, Ore.

This marks the first time that consumers can reasonably afford a super food product with such high-quality ingredients and meticulous handling.

"We realized that BõKU™ Super Food needed to be at a price that people could afford, in order for the public to benefit from its powerful attributes," Lynn M. Rollé said. "This was achieved with direct cooperation of all suppliers and farmers, and a unique direct-to-consumer business model."

Farmers grow the ingredients of BõKU™ Super Food naturally, rather than using mass production.

"We had to sell the idea to farms and suppliers that by working together in this mission to provide precious ingredients at a lower price, their investment would pay off in the long-term," Rollé said.

Enjoy this important product on a regular basis

As a physician and a homeopath, I strongly recommend to my patients that they use BõKU™ Super Food to help maintain good, vibrant health. The product has emerged as an important part of my dietary protocol, largely because BõKU™ Super Food stimulates the body's protective mechanism, making the body's pH balance more alkaline.

Largely as a result, every time a patient returns for semi-annual and annual follow-up exams, I remind them of the many benefits of taking BõKU™ Super Food—where I'm proud to serve on the company's leadership team.

Lynn M. Rollé provides an excellent service when she informs consumers that "the first and last secret of natural weight loss can be wrapped up in a single word—nutrition."

Adrezin echoes this sentiment, calling nutrition the ultimate cure and the ultimate secret to weight management.

"Nutrition provides the foundation for every living cell every organ and every metabolic chemical in your body," Adrezin said. "Nutrition defines what you are made of."

With this in mind, consumers become motivated when they discover that abundant nutrition in the blood supplies the body with the very fuel for existence. This process supplies strength, energy and vitality, while empowering the body to fight disease and illness.

"Most important, it's the reason we eat in the first place," Adrezin said. "A lack of nutrition is the bottom-line reason why we gain weight."

In fact, hunger is more than just a reason to consume food. This vital craving serves as your body's essential communication, conveying a basic need for important nutrients.

"When you eat natural, nutrient-dense foods, you satisfy your body's need for fuel," Adrezin said.

With this understood, it's important to learn about the most nutrient rich foods on earth. These include:

* Kale, spinach, beet tops and all dark green leafy vegetables
* Spirulina and chlorella
* Herbs like dandelion leaf, nettle and parsley
* Bee pollen and royal jelly
* Dark red and purple fruits and berries
* Kelp and sea plants
* Taro root, orange tomatoes, carrots, and orange vegetables

Discover how to get super nutrition

While medical professionals stress the importance of nutrition, the health industry keeps a dirty little secret—not telling you that a vast majority of vitamins and supplement products fail to work effectively.

"The body cannot break down and assimilate many supplement products," Adrezin said. "As a result, your digestive system ends up passing vitamin supplements through your system, virtually untouched!"

Thus, food provides the best way to get healthy nutrition that the body can readily absorb, particularly plants, fruits, vegetables and herbs. But most of us fail to get enough of these in our daily food intake.

Worsening matters, many industrial food farms add harmful chemicals to our fruits and vegetables in an effort to preserve crops through the long transportation process, from farms to the supermarket, and eventually to your table.

Back in the 1980s and 1990s, many people started "juicing"—liquefying plants, fruits, vegetables and herbs—in an effort to concentrate nutrients. That seemed like a great solution at the time.

"Today, we have an even better solution, one that gives you all the plant fiber as well as the nutrients and food value," Lynn M. Rollé said. "It's the green BōKU™ Super Food powder drink mix, containing pure, dried, concentrated plants in raw form."

In fact, this product is so power-packed that a single tablespoon provides the equivalent of a huge amount of fruits and vegetables. Just some of the nutrients packed within BōKU™ Super Food include:

* Spirulina and Chlorella (super nutrient-rich sea vegetables)
* Maca Root (appetite supressent and source of energy and nutrition)
* Stinging Nettle
* Horsetail Herb
* Flax Seed Meal (source of Omega-3 fatty acids and fiber)
* Wheat, Barley and Oat Grasses (nutrient-rich grasses)
* Alfalfa, Broccoli, Spinach, Kale and Dandelion Leaf Juices (help suppress appetite and provide gluten-free sources of nutrients)
* Organic fruits like Apple, Raspberry, Black Currant, Grape, and Açai (anti-oxidants)
* Kelp and other Seaweed (minerals and nutrition from the sea)
* Enzymes and Probiotic Cultures (friendly flora that help with digestion and elimination)

The probiotic cultures provide balance for your intestinal flora, reducing yeast infections, and helping with digestion and elimination. If you don't take a probiotic supplement or eat plenty of live cultures, then you should adopt the good strategy of getting this in a green drink like BōKU™ Super Food.

Use natural treatments for good colon health.

Poor dietary habits emerge as the primary cause of poor colon health, while cures remain fairly straightforward.

"The key is to eliminate or greatly reduce unhealthy foods from the diet," Adrezin said. "Foods to avoid or curtail include unsaturated fats, dairy products, excess starches and sugars, and red meat."

Among keys to getting the colon into good shape:

- **Enemas and colonics:** Colons serve as massive honeycombs that can harbor years-old waste. As gross as this might sound, several pounds of bacteria-laden fecal matter can become attached to the colon walls. This can cause chronic fatigue, flatulence, bloating, skin disorders, breathing disorders, arthritis and even constipation. Colonic cleanses help remove these wastes and intestinal parasites, restoring youthful qualities to the intestines and bowels. Meantime, hydro colon therapy and good diets can cure flatulence.
- **Probiotics**: While antibiotics fight against unwanted bacteria, probiotics serve an opposite chore—promoting the restoration of healthy bacteria within the body including intestinal flora. Acidophilus and bifidophilus serve as the most common probiotic flora. In fact, these reign as so important to the colon that it's essential to take probiotics when using antibiotics, doing a colon cleanse or undergoing chemotherapy. Probiotics enable fauna and flora to regenerate in the colon and intestines, thereby helping you ingest and absorb food. Keep in mind that antibiotics kill everything within the bacterial realm including good bacteria in your body. The lack of a healthy body flora promotes Candida yeast infections.
- **Fiber and raw foods**: Nutritionists know that fiber from raw foods can clean the intestines. Raw or lightly cooked broccoli, Brussels sprouts and cabbage often work best, while grains and seeds also prove beneficial.
- **Cholesterol connection:** Excessive cholesterol can cause gallstones in the liver and gallbladder, resulting in poor digestion and deterioration of the essential need to process fats and proteins. Unless efficiently processed into or out of the body, fats and proteins can get stuck in the colon, mucking up the works.

Coffee serves as one of the most widely used agents for enemas and colonics. In fact, coffee stimulates the lining of the colon, causing it to excrete more proficiently— while also cleaning bile ducts between the colon, liver and gallbladder. Just as important, coffee also rejuvenates the deep peristalsis, the natural movement through your entire digestive tract.

Use BōKU™ Super Cleanse for great health

For colon and intestinal health, a superior product is BōKU™ Super Cleanse. Remember that the colon works as one of our main detoxification routes. As you've learned by now, a sluggish bowel breeds toxicity that seriously and adversely affects the entire body's health. Regular bowel movements and a clean colon signal your organs are functioning at superior levels, the way nature intended.

The first step in using BōKU™ Super Cleanse involves gently and effectively moving the bowels while cleansing and detoxifying with oregano—a natural anti-bacterial substance—plus peppermint as an anti-inflammatory and soothing agent, plus fennel, rhubarb and other herbs.

This formulation also includes: Aloe Vera for soothing and healing the intestines; Napal Cactus, for fibrous bulk that helps move bowels while supporting a healthy blood sugar balance; and enzymes to help the proper functioning of the bowels.

You can take this formula on a consistent basis to help maintain regularity, heal the intestines and support healthy cholesterol levels.

The second step in this cleansing process involves pulling toxins from the digestive and intestinal tract with zeolite clay, activated charcoal, slippery elm, and other herbs. Adrezin designed this superior formulation to draw in and absorb poisons from the bowel, allowing you to eliminate them.

The cleansing product adds fibrous bulk while nourishing, soothing and lubricating the intestines as it moves through, without psyllium that can irritate and cause bloating. You also can benefit by using the cleanse for indigestion after meals; the activated charcoal and other ingredients help control acid indigestion and bloating.

Take more positive steps

After finishing your enema or colonic cleansing, you can introduce liquid chlorophyll—very healing, energizing and soothing—back into your colon. Molecularly the closest to the substance to hemoglobin in your blood cells, chlorophyll possesses superior regenerative and healing benefits.

Among colon cleanse supplement programs that also are available, most are multi-day processes that use herbs to help remove waste from the intestines. Some key ingredients used in these programs include: ground black walnut shell husk; garlic extracts; psyllium husk; bentonite clay or liquid; pau d'arco; wormwood; yellow dock; citric acid from lemon or grapefruit; cayenne pepper; and slippery elm.

"The best way to instantly lose five pounds is an enema, which you can do yourself in case you're embarrassed by a technician putting a hose in your tailpipe," Adrezin said.

Although colon work might seem embarrassing or secretive, many people who first administer enemas on themselves subsequently find no problem when such applications are administered by a professional practitioner. From our experience, hydro colon therapists perform this task in a very gentle and professional manner.

While colon therapy is great for most people, those with intestinal tumors, Chron's disease, ulcerative colitis, diverticulitis, or severe hemorrhoids should avoid enemas.

Use natural treatments to prevent colds

Benefiting consumers, BõKU™ Super Food provides important literature and Web site information on the best way to prevent colds. We recommend the strategy suggested by the company's medical experts, boosting the immune system with Vitamin C, spirulina dietary supplement and olive leaf extract, plus antioxidants from fruits and vegetables.

During cold season, or when others around you have colds, you may want to take extra Vitamin C, Echinacea with goldenseal, and Lomatium.

Since people don't always know when viruses and bacteria are making rounds, we recommend always having a cold-killing throat spray. When you feel the first signs of itching and irritation in the throat, along with an antibacterial throat spray, use the following ingredients:

- Liquid St. John's wort (50 ml)

- Liquid Echinacea (50 ml)

- Tea tree oil or propolis (a few drops)

- Grapefruit seed extract (a few drops)

For best results, mix these together and spray the solution onto your throat at the first sign of irritation. Use an eye dropper if you lack a spray tincture bottle.

In addition, pomegranate extract serves as a good topical antiviral for the throat.

And some experts prefer to apply a few drops of 3-percent hydrogen peroxide into each ear at the first signs of a cold. You can apply drops two or three times per day until symptoms disappear.

Learn to treat an existing cold

People stuck with an existing viral cold accompanied by a fever often discover that Vitamin C proves very helpful. We recommend starting with three grams, followed by one-gram increments every hour till the fever breaks.

Keep in mind that newcomers to high doses of Vitamin C may experience diarrhea, while seasoned users of this vital substance can increase doses without such side affects.

For bacterial colds that involve drippy noses, add Vitamin A or beta-carotene, and 50 milligrams of zinc Picolinate with little food. However, women who are pregnant or who may become pregnant should avoid such doses of Vitamin A

While many people automatically think of Vitamin C as a natural substance for treating common colds, they also might find themselves surprised to learn zinc also serves as a potent remedy against such illness. In fact, this substance boosts your immune system's T cells, helping to kill the cold bacteria quick and with efficiency.

Although research remains inconclusive on the affects of zinc on colds, a 2000 study that taking just 12.8 milligrams of zinc reduced the duration of cold symptoms and coughs by 50 percent, and mucus discharge by 30 percent.

Adding to the firepower against common colds, practitioners of traditional Chinese medicine prescribe ginger, considered effective by many health professionals in the West. At the first sign of a cold, steep three or four pieces of ginger in hot water to make tea before adding honey for taste. Add basil to the tea if you have chills and fever.

Among other natural treatments also considered powerful:

- **Herbs**: Speed results by adding three or four garlic, Echinacea herb and thymus glandular capsules. In addition, olive leaf extract works as a powerful antioxidant, boosting energy while decreasing recovery time from viral, bacterial and fungal infections.

- **Flu**: For colds with flu symptoms such as sore, achy muscles, mix one tablespoon of horseradish in one cup of olive oil. Let the mixture sit for

30 minutes, and then apply it as massage oil for instant relief of aching muscles.

- **Coughing**: For coughing bouts, licorice lozenges act as a natural suppressant and expectorant, enabling you to cough less—while coughing up more mucus. To break up congestion, take three or four capsules of cayenne through the day.

Benefit from natural treatments for cirrhosis

Use detoxification methods while enjoying a steady, pure diet to prevent or reverse liver disease and cirrhosis. Detoxification helps reduce symptoms of cirrhosis, while cleansing the body's natural systems. An important initial step involves a complete colon and intestinal cleanse before starting cleanses of the liver and other areas of the body.

Make sure to eat whole and organic foods that include seeds, nuts, whole grains, beans and green leafy vegetables, plus goat, soy or rice milk. All along, avoid alcohol and processed or saturated fats, including margarine and hydrogenated oils. As substitutes, use cold-processed oils such as olive oil and flaxseed oil.

For added, helpful benefit, eat foods high in amino acids and potassium. These include nuts, seeds, bananas, raisins, rice, wheat bran, kelp, Palmaria palmata, molasses, and brewer's yeast.

Meantime, you should avoid animal protein, as well as raw or undercooked fish. Juice therapy can help eliminate toxins, especially apple juice. Also try beet and carrot juices and green drinks that contain Spirulina, Chlorella and other green elements.

Herbs such as milk thistle can help treat and regulate liver cells, aiding regeneration. Other herbs, such as Picrorhiza kurroa, have a similar affect, and licorice root is often helpful. The Chinese herb bupleururn is another one to try.

Helpful nutritional supplements include Vitamin C, Vitamin E, lipoic acid, and raw liver tablets. Take regular doses of Vitamin B complex, selenium, folic acid, digestive enzymes with hydrochloric acid, and the amino acids L-carnitine, L-cysteine, L-glutathione, and L-arginine.

Other alternative therapies include acupuncture, detoxification therapy, natural hormone replacement therapy, and Traditional Chinese Medicine.

Use these supplements for chronic fatigue

Anyone who suffers from chronic fatigue knows the difficulty in boosting the body's energy. In cases of adrenal exhaustion, a variety of healthy foods or herbs support the vital glands regulating your body's energy levels. Among antiviral and food therapies to use if you're a virus causes your condition:

- Maca root

- St. John's wort

- Garlic extract

- Green tea and green tea extract

- Una de Gato, or Cat's Claw, from the Amazon (scientific name, Uncaria tomentosa).

In still other instances, low blood pressure decreases the body's energy. To augment and balance low blood pressure:

- Take an iron supplement.

- Eat Spirulina to aid in the body's absorption of minerals and help balance blood sugar levels.

- Eat foods rich in bioflavonoids, such as red grapes, green tea, bilberry, hawthorn root, and gotu kola.

- Eat antioxidant-rich foods.

Some health experts believe that chronic fatigue often results from problems based at the neuro-emotional level, even more than physical or biochemical difficulties.

Besides biological reasons, other possible causes of chronic fatigue include the loss of the will to continue, chronic hopelessness, depression, and shock or trauma.

In addition, chronic fatigue is often mistaken for Lyme disease; be sure you are tested for this if you are experiencing symptoms of chronic fatigue syndrome.

Manage your cholesterol with natural treatments

Form new disciplined eating and lifestyle habits to control your cholesterol. By adopting various habits, nutritional supplements, and foods including herbal extracts and plants, you can manage cholesterol for optimal health. Among these strategies:

- **LDL cholesterol**: To keep this under control, thereby maintaining clear arterial walls, you should add lots of garlic, soy, and lutein-rich vegetables to your diet. These foods include carrots, corn, kale, spinach, Swiss chard, collard greens and mustard greens, plus red peppers, dill, parsley, romaine lettuce, tomatoes and red, blue and purple fruits. People who use the blood-thinning drug Coumadin should consult their health providers because garlic also thins the blood.

- **Mushroom Cordyceps**: Taken in pill or tincture form, this substance reduces harmful LDL cholesterol while raising beneficial HDL cholesterol. Raised energy and inhibiting the formation of plaque in cell walls become added benefits.

- **Lipotropics**: Employed to promote the utilization of fat, these include methionine, choline and inositol.

- **Various substances**: Flaxseed oil, rapeseed oil, chia seeds, some fish and some salvia plant seeds contain vital omega-3 fatty acids. Other vital substances include Vitamin B6, non-flush niacin, chromium picolinate, pantothenic acid, red yeast and tocotrienol Vitamin E.

- **Saturated fats and omega-6 fatty acids**: Reduce your intake of these substances, contained in vegetable oils and canola, soybean, walnut, safflower and sunflower oils.

- **Oatmeal**: High-fiber foods like this also help lower potentially harmful LDL cholesterol. Your body reaps more benefits from whole grains rather than refined grains; whole grains play a role in preventing diabetes and obesity.

- **Red wine**: Drink one glass each night to benefit from its powerful polyphenols that inhibit the oxidation of LDL cholesterol. The many antioxidants and bioflavonoids in red wine add additional health improvements.

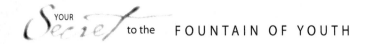

APPENDIX 3

PHYSICIAN REFERRAL RESOURCES

The following represents an incomplete list of more than an estimated 20,000 physicians who regularly prescribe human growth hormone for the purpose of age-related growth hormone deficiency (GHD) syndrome.

Many of these "cutting edge" physicians prefer to remain "under the radar," despite the fact that the "not guilty verdict" of James W. Forsythe, M.D., H.M.D., now gives them legal precedent to practice good medicine. These physicians are listed by geographical regions for the reader's convenience.

LISTED STATES	REGION
Arizona	Southwestern United States
California	West Coast
Colorado	Mountain States
Connecticut	Mid-Atlantic United States
Florida	Southeastern United States
Georgia	Southeastern United States
Idaho	Great Basin Region
Illinois	Midwestern United States
Indiana	Midwestern United States
Maryland	Mid-Atlantic United States
Massachusetts	Northeastern United States
Michigan	Midwestern United States
Minnesota	Midwestern United States
Nevada	Great Basin Region
New York	Northeastern United States
New Jersey	Mid-Atlantic United States
North Carolina	Southeastern United States
Pennsylvania	Mid-Atlantic United States
Tennessee	Midwestern United States
Texas	Southwestern United States

Utah	Mountain States
Vermont	Northeastern United States
Virginia	Mid-Atlantic United States
Washington	Great Basin Region
Wisconsin	Midwestern United States

GREAT BASIN REGION

IDAHO:
> Post Falls

> > Paul Brillhart, M.D.
> > (208) 773-1311
> > www.drpaulbrillhart.com

NEVADA:
> Carson City

> > Frank Shallenberger, M.D., H.M.D.
> > (775) 884-3990

> Las Vegas

> > Julie Garcia, M.D.
> > (702) 870-0058

> > Robert Milne, M.D.
> > (702) 385-1393

> > Fuller Royal, M.D.
> > (702) 732-1400

> Reno

> > James W. Forsythe, M.D., H.M.D.
> > Earlene M. Forsythe, A.P.N.
> > (775) 827-0707
> > www.drforsythe.com

WASHINGTON:
> Bellingham

Andrew Pauli, M.D.
(360) 527-9785

MID-ATLANTIC UNITED STATES

CONNECTICUT:
Manchester

Stephen Sinatra, M.D.
(860) 643-5101

MARYLAND:
Baltimore

Dean Kane, M.D.
(410) 602-3322

B. Rothstein, D.O.
(410) 484-2121

NEW JERSEY:
Cherry Hill

Allan Magaziner, M.D.
(856) 424-8222
www.drmagaziner.com

Vijay Vijh, M.D.
(856) 489-0505

Shrewsbury

Neil Rosen, M.D.
(732) 219-0895

Trenton

Initiaz Ahmad, M.D.

(609) 890-2966

PENNSYLVANIA:
Pittsburgh

Brenda McMahon, M.D.
(412) 487-8638

VIRGINIA:
Arlington

Denise Bruner, M.D.
(703) 558-4949

Virginia Beach

Jennifer Krup, M.D.
(757) 306-4300

MIDWESTERN UNITED STATES

ILLINOIS:
Chicago:

Paul Savage, M.D.
(866) 535-2563
www.bodylogicmd.com

John Zaborowski, M.D.
(847) 291-4148

Libertyville

Craig Dean, M.D.
(847) 367-6347

INDIANA:
Goshen

Tammy Born, M.D.
www.bornclinic.com

Indianapolis

Linda Spencer, M.D.
(317) 298-3850
www.complementaryfamilymedicalcare.com

Lafayette

Charles Turner, M.D.
(765) 471-1100
www.charlesturnermd.com

MICHIGAN:
Canton

Pamela Smith, M.D.
(734) 398-7522

Detroit

Cynthia Shelby-Lane, M.D.
(800) 436-9777

Grand Rapids

Tammy Born, M.D.
(616) 656-3700
www.bornclinic.com

Southfield:

Edward Lichten, M.D.
(248) 358-3433

West Bloomfield

David Brownstein, M.D.

(248) 851-1600

MINNESOTA:
Edina

Khalid Mahmud, M.D.
(952) 943-1529

TENNESSEE:
Bristol

David Marden, D.O.
(423) 844-4925

WISCONSIN:
Waukesha

James Nagel, M.D.
(262) 542-0860

MOUNTAIN STATES

COLORADO:
Denver

Peter Hanson, M.D.
(303) 733-2521
www.peterhansonmd.com

UTAH:
St. George

Gordon Reynolds, M.D.
(435) 628-8060

NORTHEASTERN UNITED STATES

MASSACHUSETTS:
Brookline

Alan Altman, M.D.
(617) 232-0262

NEW YORK:
New York

Eric Braverman, M.D.
(212) 213-6188

Rashmi Gulati
(212) 794-4466
www.patientsmedical.com

Ronald Hoffman, M.D.
(212) 779-1744
www.drhoffman.com

Alexander Kulice, M.D.
(212) 838-8265
www.ostrow.medem.com

Richard Linchitz, M.D.
(212) 252-1942
www.metropolitanwellness.com

Jeffrey Morrison, M.D.
(212) 989-9828
www.themorrisoncenter.com

John Salerno, M.D.
(212) 582-1700

www.salernocenter.com

Erika Schwartz, M.D.
(212) 873-3420

Port Washington
Thomas Lodi, M.D.
(516) 883-6771

Rhinebeck

Steven Bock, M.D.
(845) 876-7082
www.rhinebeckhealth.com

VERMONT:
New Chapter
Paul Schulick, M.D.
(802) 257-9345
www.new-chapter.info

SOUTHEASTERN UNITED STATES

FLORIDA:
Boca Raton
Gary Brandwein, D.O.
(954) 396-3908

Lauderhill

Herbert Slavin, M.D.
(954) 748-4991

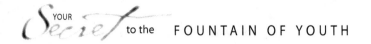 to the FOUNTAIN OF YOUTH

Sarasota
Robert Carlson, M.D.
(941) 955-1815
www.preventaging.org

GEORGIA:
Alpharetta
Daniela Paunesky, M.D.
(770) 777-7707

Stockbridge
Frank McCafferty, M.D.
(770) 506-0087

NORTH CAROLINA:
Greensboro
Larry Webster, M.D.
(336) 272-2030
www.lwebster.com

SOUTHWESTERN UNITED STATES

ARIZONA:
Tucson
Dharma Khalsa, M.D.
(520) 749-8374

Daniel Mihalyi, M.D.
(520) 742-1585

Sun City
Alan Miles, M.D.

(623) 974-2226

TEXAS:

Bulverde

Donna Becker, D.O.

Dallas

Clark Ridley, M.D.
(214) 303-1888
www.lifespanmedicine.com

Houston

Gurney Pearsall, M.D.
(713) 522-4037

Theodore Piliszek, M.D.
(281) 469-4156

The Woodlands

Garth Denyer, M.D.
(281) 367-1414

Weatherford

Ronald McDaniel, D.O.
(817) 599-4301

Wimberly

Lane Sebring, M.D.
(512) 847-5618

WEST COAST

CALIFORNIA:
Beverly Hills

Jennifer Berman, M.D.
(310) 432-6644

Cathie Lippman, M.D.
(310) 289-8430

Gary London, M.D.
(310) 207-4500

Prabin Mishra, M.D.
(310) 247-8577

Uzzi Reiss, M.D.
(310) 474-1945

Bishop

David Greene, M.D.
(760) 873-8982

Burlingame

Tedde Rinker, D.O.
(650) 259-9500

Encino

Mark Gordon, M.D.
(818) 990-1166

Fresno

Narges Mazj, M.D.
(559) 433-9170

Los Angeles

Michael Galitzer, M.D.
(800) 392-2623

Hans Gruenn, M.D.
(310) 966-9194

Ann Pretre, M.D.
(310) 839-1510

Joseph Sciabbarrasi, M.D.
(310) 268-8466

Michael P. Wai Lam, M.D.
(213) 383-0105

Los Gatos

Phillip Lee Miller, M.D.
(408) 358-8855

Newport Beach

Catherine Arvantely, M.D.
(949) 660-1399

Orange

Gary Ruelas, M.D.
(714) 771-2880

Pasadena

Maria Sulindro, M.D.
(626) 403-6200

Redding

Robert Greene, M.D.
(530) 244-9052

San Diego

Joseph Filbeck, M.D.
(848) 457-5700

Ron Rothenberg, M.D.
(800) 943-3331

Santa Barbara

Robert Mathis, M.D.
(805) 569-7100

Julie Taguchi, M.D.
(805) 681-7500

Duncan Turner, M.D.
(805) 682-6340

Santa Monica

David Allen, M.D.
(310) 966-9194

Prudence Hall, M.D.
(310) 458-7979

Santee

Stephen Center, M.D.
(858) 273-5757

Upland

Wendy Miller Rashidi, M.D.

(909) 982-4000

<u>Woodland Hills</u>

Jerel Tilton, M.D.
(818) 704-5500

Authors' contact information

James W. Forsthe, M.D., H.M.D.

Century Wellness Clinic

Toll Free: (877-789-0707)

521 Hammill Lane, Reno, NV 89511

www.drforsythe.com

Voice: 775-827-0707   Fax: 775-827-1006

CPSIA information can be obtained
at www.ICGtesting.com
Printed in the USA
LVHW052240100719
623748LV00022B/893/P